Emergency reference

Angina 125

Animal bites. 21

Back injuries. 15

Bee stings. 26

Bites: animal 21
     human .25
     insect 28
     marine life 30
     snake 22

Bleeding. 35

Blisters 150

Blocked airway 78

Breathing problems. 65

Broken: arm 50
     collarbone 48
     back 15
     bone 46
     elbow .56
     hip. 58
     jaw. 120
     leg. 58
     neck 15
     nose .134
     shoulder 48
     tooth .129

Bruises 87

Burns. 69

Cat bites. 25

Charleyhorse 131

Chemical: burns 74
     in the eye 107
     swallowed 136

Chest: pain. 123
     injury. .75

Chills. 112

Choking. 77

Choking during convulsions 94

Cleaning solvents: in the eye 107
     swallowed. 136

Convulsions 93

Concussions 120

Contractions (during pregnancy). 140

Cramps: during pregnancy. 140
     muscle 131

Croup 68

Cuts (minor). 84

Dehydration. 156

Diarrhea. 158

Dislocations 45

Dizziness. 161

Dog bites 25

Drowning 164

Drug overdose 135

Ear problems 97

Electric: burns .72
     shock .99

Eye injuries 103

Exposure: cold 112
     heat .110

Fainting. 161

Fever 115

Fishhook. 92

Fits 93

Frostbite 113

Gagging. 77

Headache 119

Head injuries .119

Heart attack. .123

Heat exhaustion 110

Heatstroke 110

Heimlich Maneuver 79

Hyperventilation 66

Hypothermia .112

Insect bites. 28

Intestinal pain .153

Jelly fish stings. 32

Knee injuries 60

Mosquito bites .28

Mouth injuries. 127

Muscle: cramps 131
     strains 131

Nausea. 153

Neck injuries 15

Nose: foreign objects. 134
     injuries 134

Nosebleeds 42

Passing out. 160

Pesticides: in the eye 107
     swallowed 136

Poison: in the eye 107
     on the skin 151
     swallowed 136

Pregnancy complications. 139

Rash: with fever. 118
     allergic, etc.. 148

Rescue: general 141
     ice. 168
     live electric current 72
     smoke or fumes 138
     water 164

Scorpion stings 26

Skin problems 147

Seizures 93

Shortness of breath 66

Smoke inhalation. 138

Snake bites. 22

Splinters 88

Spotting (during pregnancy) 140

Sprains: back. 46
     neck. .46
     other. .45

Stings: insects .28
     marine-life 30

Stomach pain 154

Stroke 94

Sunburn 70

Sunstroke 110

Swallowed objects 82

Throwing up .156

Tightness in the chest. 123

Tooth loss (sudden) 129

Unconsciousness 159

Vomiting. 156

Water accidents 163

THE
Johnson & Johnson
FIRST AID BOOK

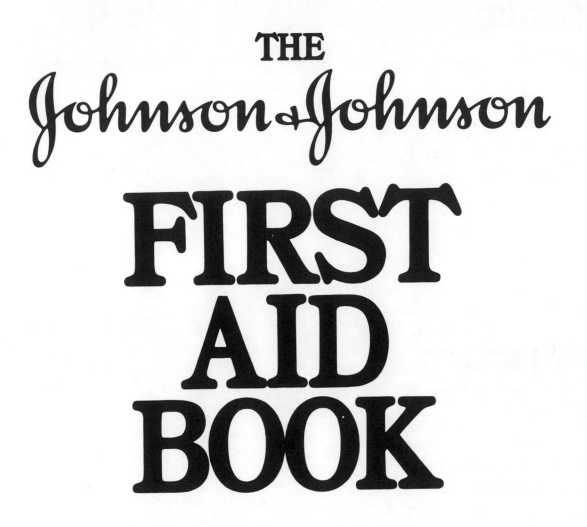

Stephen N. Rosenberg, M.D.

with the cooperation and medical review of
The College of Physicians & Surgeons of Columbia University and
The Section of Emergency Services,
University of Michigan Medical School

WARNER BOOKS

A Warner Communications Company

Credits

Editor / Reid Boates

Concept and Art Direction / UNION GRAPHIK INC.

Design / Leah Turell

Illustrations / Werner Abken

Editorial Assistant / Niza Leichtman-Davidson, PhD

Warner Books, Inc., 666 Fifth Avenue, New York, NY 10103

A Warner Communications Company

Printed in the United States of America

10 9 8 7

Acknowledgments

The authors and publishers are extremely grateful to the following for their meticulous review, comments, and contributions during the development of this book.

Thomas Q. Morris, M.D.
Professor of Clinical Medicine
College of Physicians and Surgeons of Columbia University
President, The Presbyterian Hospital in the City of New York

Kenneth C. Fine, M.D.
Assistant Professor of Clinical Medicine
College of Physicians and Surgeons of Columbia University
Director of Combined Emergency Services at The Presbyterian
    Hospital in the City of New York

Richard E. Burney, M.D.
Associate Professor of Surgery
Sections of Emergency Services and General Surgery
University of Michigan Medical School

James R. Mackenzie, M.D.
Associate Professor of Surgery
Sections of Emergency Services and General Surgery
University of Michigan Medical School

Gerald P. Hodge
Professor, Postgraduate Medicine and Health Professions—
    Education
Professor, School of Art
Director, Graduate Program in Medical and Biological Illustration
University of Michigan

Contents

Introduction   8
    How to assess an emergency   9
    How to take a pulse   10
    Emotional factors in first aid   12
    Preparation for emergencies   13
Back & Neck Injuries   15
Bites & Stings   21
Bleeding   35
Breaks, Sprains & Dislocations   45
Breathing Problems   65
Burns   69
Chest Injuries   75
Choking & Swallowed Objects   77
Common Injuries (Soft Tissue Injuries)   83
Convulsions (Seizures, Fits)   93
Ear Problems   97
Electric Shock   99
Eye Injuries   103
Exposure to Heat & Cold   109

Fever   115
Head Injuries   119
Heart Attack & Chest Pain   123
Mouth Injuries   127
Muscle Cramps & Strains   131
Nose Injuries & Foreign Objects in the Nose   133
Poisoning & Drug Overdose   135
Pregnancy Complications   139
Rescue in Emergencies   141
Skin Problems: Rashes, Blisters & Contact Poisons 147
Stomach & Intestinal Problems   153
Unconsciousness & Fainting (Unrelated to Injury) 159
Water Accidents: Water & Ice Rescue   163
Family Emergency Chart   173

Introduction

IN AN EMERGENCY, TURN IMMEDIATELY TO THE "EMERGENCY REFERENCE" PAGE AT THE VERY FRONT OF THIS BOOK.

This book has been designed to give you clear, complete, and systematic directions—quickly—for any situation requiring first aid. It is not only an authoritative guide to emergency care; it also has a number of unique features that make it ideal for on-the-spot use:

First, the book stays open when it is laid flat, so that both of your hands are free for whatever has to be done. Just as important, all the information you need to handle a given emergency situation is presented—in step-by-step words and illustrations—on a single page or two facing pages. Everything you need to know is right in front of you, and the need to turn to other parts of the book is kept to an absolute minimum. Instructions that apply to a wide variety of situations (such as "Do not move a person with a possible broken neck") are repeated whenever applicable to ensure that every section of the book is self-contained.

Cross-references to other parts of the book are included to make sure that you have not turned to an inappropriate chapter (*Mouth Injuries*, for example, instead of *Head Injuries: Skull & Scalp*) and to remind you of related problems and special cases (a victim of *Drowning* may also have *Back & Neck Injuries*).

Other features, described in detail below, will help you use this book quickly and effectively in an emergency and will also give you a solid grounding in the reasons for first aid and the methods of emergency care. Take the time to familiarize yourself with these features, and you'll know how to get the information you need when the unexpected occurs. We'll illustrate with an example.

Suppose a friend arrives at your home for dinner. He takes a seat in your living room while you check on a dish in the oven. When you return from the kitchen, your friend is breathing rapidly, looks frightened, and says he can't catch his breath. What should you do?

Finding the right section

You take this book down from your bookshelf. Just inside the front cover is a complete alphabetical listing, in everyday English, of major and minor emergencies. In this case, you'd see that *Breathing Problems* is obviously the chapter you want. Open immediately to the cited page. (There is also a thorough *Index* at the back of the book, but you should rarely need it in an emergency. It is primarily for use in finding details, such as general information regarding hyperventilation.)

What you open to (as with all chapters) is a *chapter cover page*, where an *Overview* gives a brief summary of the chapter and the most important general information. In *Breathing Problems*, for example, it points out the importance of calming down any person who is having difficulty breathing. The chapter cover page also lists the sections in the chapter (with page numbers) and further describes the contents of each section. The appropriate entry here says, "*Shortness of breath:* What to do for a person who is breathing rapidly and feels 'out of breath.'" You turn to that section.

Important—read first

Each section begins with a box at the upper left, headed: *Important—read first*. It lists all the crucial things to do (for shortness of breath, for example, you are told to check for signs of possible heart disease) and the significant dangers to be avoided—what *not* to do. It gives you at a glance all the important do's and don'ts to keep in mind when you are performing the sequential steps of first aid.

General instructions—to help you choose the right alternative

In many emergency situations, you will have to choose among several first-aid possibilities depending on conditions—such as whether a person is conscious or unconscious or, with shortness of breath, whether the signs of heart disease are present or absent. Just below the *Important—read first* box, instructions are provided to help you sort out priorities so that you can start treatment at the most useful point and avoid procedures that are unnecessary or harmful.

Doctor's comments

At the bottom of the left-hand page are *Doctor's comments*. These explain the why and wherefores of the situation—how shortness of breath, for example, can cause such seemingly unrelated symptoms as tingling of the hands and feet, and why breathing into a bag will bring relief. These comments, while not part of the actual instructions, will give you a more complete understanding of the condition in question and of first-aid procedures. When there is time, you will want to read them to learn; but in an emergency, they can wait until the situation is under control.

The first-aid steps

Most of each section is devoted to step-by-step instructions for first aid. The "Shortness of breath" section gives, first, 5 steps for all shortness of breath. Detailed illustrations combine with the instructions for quick and accurate understanding by the reader.

When giving first aid, you will often have to work with whatever materials are available. For shortness of breath, you'd look for a paper bag or a bowl, or have the person use his own cupped hands. This particular choice is a minor one, but decisions among alternatives are often crucial in emergencies. When you must immobilize a fracture, the procedure varies depending on whether or not materials for splints are available. When an injured person must be carried, the choice of method depends, among other factors, on the number of rescuers and the distance to be traveled. To the extent possible, the instructions in this book prepare you for all of these situations.

Read ahead of time

The procedures presented in this book have been chosen because they are effective and the most practical for the people who are the most likely to use them: nonprofessional first-aiders. Follow the directions carefully, as calmly and gently as possible, and you could save a life. Learn the steps and principles of first aid *ahead of time*, and you're much more likely to be confident, level-headed, and helpful in an emergency.

Family emergency chart

Finally, the book concludes with a *Family emergency chart* which should be filled out carefully and fully as soon as possible. Properly completed, this chart will be an invaluable source of accurate information in the event of emergency.

How to assess an emergency

One of the most important tools in first aid is the technique called cardiopulmonary resuscitation (CPR). If you do not know CPR, the authors urge you to take a course. *You cannot learn proper CPR techniques from a book.* This specialized training, available from your local American Red Cross chapter and other agencies, is essential in treating persons with cardiac arrest, acute airway obstruction, and respiratory distress. As you read this book, it will become apparent that knowing this lifesaving technique will enhance your ability to carry out first aid treatments.

If you do not know where to find classes in CPR, call your local Red Cross chapter or contact the American Heart Association.

Know the priorities—what to do first, next, and so forth

The most stressful experiences in first aid occur when you don't know what to do first. Several people involved in an accident may all require help; an accident victim may have more than one injury; or the nature of someone's injury or illness may be unclear, as with a child too young to explain or an adult who is unconscious, panicky, or confused. In any of these situations, you can sort things out appropriately by observing these priorities:

1. Ask for help
Shout for help before you do anything else. If others at the scene of an accident can assist you, you can treat several people or injuries at once, or someone else can phone for an ambulance while you give first aid. If you are trained in lifesaving techniques such as cardiopulmonary resuscitation, don't spend time phoning or looking for help until after you have given initial care for life-threatening emergencies that will not wait.

2. Check for dangers to yourself
Avoid becoming a second victim. Is there an electric hazard in the area? Gas, smoke, or fumes? Water or thin ice? A danger of falling? A violent individual? You must plan to avoid these hazards before you can help someone else. *If there are hazards, call for help.*

3. Look for dangers to the injured person
If external dangers are present, you must move an injured or sick person to safety, if this does not endanger you as well. If the person is in the path of oncoming traffic, in a burning auto or a building that may collapse, plan to move him if you can do so without jeopardizing your own safety. If at all possible, give brief first aid for the most urgent conditions.

Other dangers, inherent in the injury, are reasons for *not* moving the person. For example, if at all possible, you should not move someone with a possible back or neck injury. Protect the victim as much as possible. Do not move unless *absolutely* necessary.

4. If you have had formal CPR training, check for and treat immediate threats to life.
First, check breathing. If a person is not breathing or cannot breathe because of choking *and you are trained in CPR,* re-start his respiration before doing anything else. Next, check the pulse. If a person is breathing, he will always have a heartbeat; but if he is not breathing,

his heart may have stopped as well. If you are trained in CPR attempt to resuscitate the victim. If not, call for help.

The third immediate threat to life is severe bleeding. Control bleeding (see page 35) right after you've checked breathing and pulse.

There is another emergency in which seconds count: chemical burns (see page 74). Even though most chemical burns are not immediately life-threatening, rapid action can prevent blindness or extensive injury.

5. Seek medical assistance
If you are alone with an injured or sick person and have not been able to summon help, you should at this point take a few minutes to telephone 911 or Operator or find someone else who can call for assistance. For any serious injury or illness, the best assistance you can summon is an ambulance staff of trained emergency medical technicians ("EMTs"), or paramedics, who can give on-the-spot care and ensure safe movement of the person.

It is important to know under what circumstances you should call for an ambulance, how to call for an ambulance, and what to do until the ambulance arrives.

A. Know whether there is an EMT system or emergency phone number in your area. Keep this phone number handy.

B. Dial 911, operator, or your emergency phone number for any of the following problems: cardiac distress, respiratory distress, poisonings, major trauma, unconsciousness, altered mental status, or paralysis. Emergency medical technicians can help and if necessary perform rescues in these situations.

C. Be sure to say, **"This is a medical emergency."**
Give:
- [ ] the phone number from which you are calling
- [ ] your location and how to find it
- [ ] the circumstances—what is the nature of the problem or complaint
- [ ] your name

This helps dispatch an ambulance or rescue vehicle quickly to the scene.

6. Treat other urgent conditions
The following list includes serious conditions for which care should be given as soon as possible—before an ambulance arrives. They are listed in rough priority order (in case you must deal with two or more of them in sequence), but each can vary in severity and move up or down on the list:

- [ ] Poisoning or drug overdose
- [ ] Heatstroke
- [ ] Moderate bleeding
- [ ] Poisonous bites or stings
- [ ] Hypothermia (lowered body temperature)
- [ ] Heart attack
- [ ] Broken bones, sprains, or dislocations
- [ ] Eye injuries

How to take a pulse

7. Treat or prevent shock

When any severe illness or injury overwhelms the body's defenses, shock may set in. Shock is essentially a sudden drop in blood pressure so severe that the brain and other vital organs do not receive the blood flow they need. It can be treated successfully only after the condition causing it (bleeding, poisoning, etc.) has been brought under control. It is important to recognize and treat shock to prevent further cardiorespiratory problems. While waiting for medical help you can raise the victim's legs and turn him on his side if he is vomiting. If shock is associated with an accident, assume the victim has neck or back injuries and use a "log roll" (see page 19) to keep his neck and back stable while turning him on his side.

8. Treat less urgent conditions

Once the above conditions, injuries, or illnesses have been controlled, (or if none is present), care for other conditions as described in this book.

In a variety of first-aid situations, you will need to take a pulse. Be sure you know the proper technique and what a normal pulse feels like.

1. Technique

The best way to learn is to check your own pulse. Do it now. Place the tips of your index, middle and ring fingers on the inside surface of your other arm, just above the wrist joint. (Never feel for pulse with your thumb. There is a faint pulse in your thumb itself, and you may feel that rather than the pulse you are checking for.) Find the hard bone on the edge of the forearm at the wrist crease below the thumb. Slide your fingers toward the soft underside of the wrist, stopping before your fingers reach the bundle of firm tendons running down the middle of the forearm, and press firmly. You probably won't feel anything if you don't press at all; you will stop the pulse if you press too hard.

You are now feeling a normal pulse. Continue to check your own pulse, examining its rate, strength, and regularity.

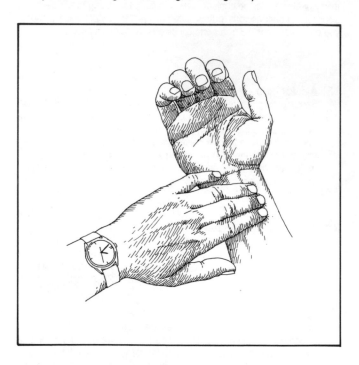

2. Rate

To measure your pulse rate, you need to have a clock or watch with a second hand (or digital seconds). The watch should be on the wrist of the hand that is doing the feeling. Count the number of pulse beats in a full minute. (When you are in a hurry, count beats for 15 seconds and multiply by 4.)

The average pulse rate for a relaxed adult is 70 to 72 beats per minute, but perfectly normal adults have rates as low as 60 and as high as 90. Newborn infants have normal resting pulse rates of about 120 per minute, which gradually slow as they get older.

Everyone's pulse speeds up with exercise or excitement, but a very rapid pulse when at rest may be an important sign in first-aid situations. A rapid pulse, for example, occurs in shock; during an asthma attack, a pulse rate of 120 or more is a sign of severe strain, requiring medical care.

3. Strength
Feel the normal strength of your own pulse.

A person in shock from bleeding or diabetic coma has a pulse that is weak and hard to feel. A weak or absent pulse in the arm should lead to examination at another site (other arm, neck). A very weak or absent pulse in just one limb means that local blood flow has been cut off. If you have just tied on a bandage to control bleeding or to hold a splint in place, loosen it.

If you check the pulse at the neck or on an uninjured, unbandaged limb and it appears to be absent, it may be too weak for you to feel, or the person's heart may have stopped beating. If he is not breathing either, assume the latter and begin CPR if you are properly trained. Otherwise, call for help.

4. Regularity
Many healthy people have some respiratory variation in their heartbeats, often influenced by their breathing. While checking your own pulse, breathe in and out slowly and very deeply a few times. You may notice a quickening of the pulse during each inward breath and a slowing during each exhalation. It may also be normal for a "skipped beat" to occur once every few minutes. Irregularity more dramatic, frequent or chaotic than these normal variations may be a sign of heart disease.

5. Location
Besides the wrist, there are two other important sites for pulse taking. You should practice them all on yourself. Use the same technique of firm but gentle pressure with the tips of three fingers.

Neck:
First place your fingertips on the Adam's apple. Then move them toward the side of the neck until you reach the groove between the windpipe and the muscles. This is the most convenient pulse to check while giving mouth-to-mouth respiration to an adult or child. When other pulses are too weak to feel, this one is often the strongest.

Upper Arm:
Feel between the muscles on the inner side of the upper arm, halfway between the shoulder and elbow. This is the easiest pulse to check while giving mouth-to-mouth respiration to a baby.

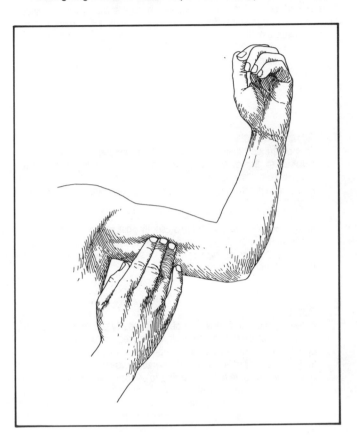

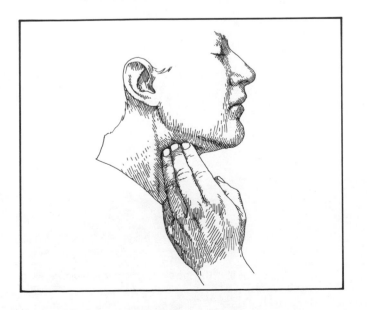

Emotional factors in first aid

Dealing with emotional reactions at the scene of an accident may be more important—and more difficult—than treating physical injuries. People who have been injured, those lucky enough to have escaped unharmed, and even bystanders may exhibit behavior that endangers them and others and makes it difficult to render first aid. Studies of natural disasters and large-scale accidents have identified five general types of psychological reaction: normal anxiety, panic, depression, hyperactivity, and bodily dysfunction. You may also see these symptoms in family members when a person has been injured or has become suddenly and dramatically ill.

1. Normal Anxiety

After a serious accident, it is normal for witnesses as well as those involved to display some signs of anxiety such as trembling, weakness, sweating, rapid breathing, a pounding heartbeat, nausea (perhaps with vomiting), mild diarrhea, frequent urination, and confusion.

In most people, these symptoms usually pass without assistance, but it is helpful to reassure the anxious person, provide some useful activity to occupy him, and watch him to be sure that he is gradually gaining—not losing—composure.

2. Panic

A person in a panic may rush about aimlessly or run away from the scene with untreated injuries and without regard for traffic and other dangers. Uncontrolled weeping is common. Act quickly: Panic is contagious. Gently but firmly, take the person away from others until he is under control. Give him something to eat or drink, preferably something warm. If he is a smoker (and there is nothing flammable around) a cigarette may calm him down. Encourage him to talk. If necessary, get help to prevent him from harming himself, but do not. use physical restraint, slap him, or throw water on him.

3. Depression

A depressed person may stand or sit motionless or walk about slowly and aimlessly, apparently unaware of his surroundings. He is not likely to talk except to respond to questions with one or two words. His expression may be vacant or dazed.

Try to establish contact gently by discussing the accident or injury and asking him to tell you about it and about his feelings. Don't express pity, but don't be harsh by telling him to "Snap out of it." Give him something warm to eat or drink and a task to perform: but not a crucial one, since he may not follow through without supervision.

4. Hyperactivity

Someone with a minor injury or an uninjured person who suffers a "close call" may become hyperactive. He will start talking rapidly, arguing or joking, jumping from one first-aid activity to another and interfering with efforts to help the seriously injured.

Don't argue with the hyperactive person. Let him talk it out, give him something to eat, if he has no injuries that could be aggravated by exercise, let him work off his excess energy in some useful physical task.

5. Bodily dysfunction

Some extremely distraught people will convert their anxiety into physical symptoms, such as prolonged vomiting or an inability to speak, see or move some part of the body. This reaction is easily confused with physical illness or injury.

Treat the symptoms as if they were real: You probably won't be sure anyway, so this is the safest course. Don't ridicule what you believe to be "fake" symptoms: They are very real to the person involved, and he won't welcome the assurance that "It's all in your mind." If possible, involve the person in the care of someone else whom you can describe as "even more severely injured." This may relieve his focus on his own condition.

Preparation for emergencies

A. Use this book to learn and practice first aid

To increase your confidence when an emergency arises, it will be helpful to read this book all the way through at your leisure. When a friend or family member does need your help, a level head—gained through understanding and competence—will be your most valuable piece of first-aid equipment.

Think about the reasons for each first-aid procedure as explained in the steps and *Doctor's comments*. A technique is easier to remember when it is understood and not seen as a mysterious set of arbitrary instructions.

Review the material on taking a pulse a few times if it is new to you. If you are unfamiliar with thermometers, look over the instructions for their use in the chapter on *Fever*.

You may want to practice some actual first-aid procedures. Two in particular are worth rehearsing: cardiopulmonary resuscitation (CPR) and first aid for choking. These procedures are a bit complex, and they need to be applied quickly in an emergency. Formal training in CPR is *mandatory*. It should *not be practiced* on family or friends. If you are trained in CPR, be gentle when you rehearse the procedure. Only pretend to give full chest compressions, back blows, and abdominal thrusts (the Heimlich maneuver); do not apply the force you would use in a real emergency.

If practicing these first-aid methods interests you and you want to go even further in preparing yourself for emergencies, you should sign up for courses sponsored by your local chapter of the American National Red Cross. Instruction is usually available in basic and advanced first aid, CPR, and lifesaving and water safety.

B. Emergency identification

If you or a family member have any serious medical condition or allergy, having this information with you at all times could save your life. If you ever are unconscious or otherwise unable to speak to rescuers, some form of emergency identification will provide critical clues, especially for someone with epilepsy, diabetes, hemophilia, or an allergy to insect stings or any medication. Ask your doctor how to order an identification necklace or bracelet, or make your own I.D. card for your wallet or pocketbook. Include your name, address, phone number, whom to contact in emergencies, what you are allergic to, your medical conditions, the medications you take, and the name and phone number of the doctor who has your medical records. If you know your blood type, list it as well.

C. Driving to the emergency service

If you have a car, be sure that you know the shortest route to the nearest 24-hour hospital emergency department. Drive there from your home the next chance you have, and do it again every year or so, just in case a street has been changed to one-way or the emergency entrance has been moved to another side of the hospital.

D. First-aid kits

Put together some basic first-aid supplies in a sturdy carton and place it in a convenient location in your home. Be sure the box is out of the reach of children. From time to time check your supplies against the list below, and replace anything that has been used:

- ☐ Sterile gauze pads, individually wrapped
- ☐ BAND-AID® brand adhesive bandages in assorted shapes and sizes
- ☐ Roll of gauze bandage
- ☐ Cravats and elastic bandages
- ☐ Adhesive tape
- ☐ Scissors
- ☐ Absorbent cotton or cotton balls
- ☐ Cotton-tipped swabs
- ☐ Oral and rectal thermometers
- ☐ Petroleum jelly for the rectal thermometer
- ☐ Syrup of Ipecac to induce vomiting
- ☐ Antihistamines (e.g. Sudafed, Benedryl)
- ☐ Peptobismol or Kaopectate for diarrhea
- ☐ Antibiotic ointments
- ☐ Measuring spoon
- ☐ Tweezers
- ☐ Safety pins
- ☐ Sharp needle
- ☐ Calamine lotion
- ☐ Paper clip
- ☐ After-bite for neutralizing bee stings
- ☐ Single-edged razor blades or sharp penknife

A similar kit should be in the trunk of your car, on your boat, or in your recreational vehicle (along with an extra copy of this book). In addition, you will need a few items in your vehicle that would normally be handy around the house:

- ☐ Flashlight
- ☐ Pad and pen or pencil
- ☐ Soap
- ☐ Cravats or triangular bandages or clean sheet for making bandages and slings
- ☐ Towel for padding splints
- ☐ Blanket for warmth in shock or hypothermia
- ☐ Paper cups
- ☐ Baby oil
- ☐ If you do any camping, add a snakebite kit.
- ☐ If anyone in the family has special needs, be sure they are provided for (a spare inhaler for asthma, extra medication for any chronic illness).

E. Family emergency chart

Take a few minutes right now to fill out the chart on the inside of the back cover for each member of your household.

If your children are sometimes at home with a babysitter, be sure he or she knows where this book and the chart are.

When listing the telephone number for an ambulance service, be sure that it is one that staffs its vehicles with trained emergency medical technicians (EMTs) or paramedics who can give on-the-spot care. (Most public and some private ambulance services have EMTs, but some private ambulance companies do not.)

Back & Neck
Injuries

overview:

The history of an injury will indicate possible damage to the back or neck. Determine possible back or neck injury by asking "what happened, how did it happen?" Is the person lying at the bottom of the stairs, has he been thrown from a car, etc.? If the circumstances suggest it, provide first aid keeping in mind that there is a suspected back or neck injury.

The most important step in first aid for a known or suspected back or neck injury is immobilization of the injured person to prevent spinal cord damage. Follow instructions under **How to Immobilize.**

If—and only if—someone with a suspected back or neck injury
□ is endangered by fire or another immediate threat to life,
   OR
□ has no pulse,
   OR
□ is not breathing,
   OR
□ is vomiting,
follow instructions under **When and How to Move Someone** on the following pages.

17 **How to immobilize**

18-19 **When and How to Move Someone with a Possible Back or Neck Injury** Signs of possible injury. When—and only when— to move the person. How to avoid further injury when moving.

Back & Neck Injuries
How to immobilize

Important—read first:

Do not move the person or let him move unless his life is threatened by an immediate danger.

Do not twist or bend the injured person's back, neck, or head.

To prevent shock, cover the person lightly to keep him warm, but do not change his position.

Seek medical assistance immediately.

If the injured person has a pulse, has no trouble breathing, is in no immediate danger from fire or other hazard, and is not vomiting:

1. Immobilize him in the exact position in which he was found by placing rolled towels, blankets, newspaper, or clothing next to his head, neck, and torso. Heavy handbags make especially good supports. Secure towels, clothing, and other light materials in place with heavy objects such as stones, bricks, etc.

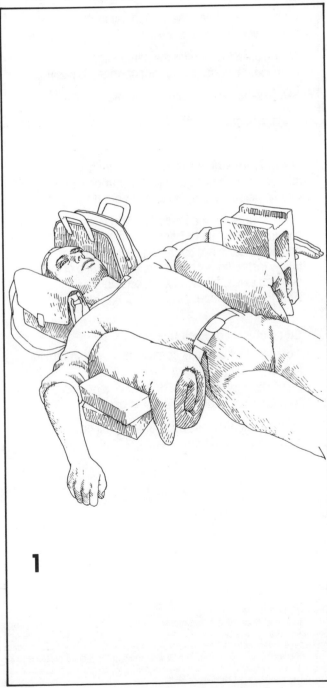

1

Doctor's comments:
Many vertebral fractures do not cause spinal-cord injury. Immobilizing the person, moving him gently, correctly, and only when absolutely necessary can prevent cord damage. When injury involves only the vertebral bones, they usually heal well.

Back & Neck Injuries

When and how to move someone with a possible back or neck injury

Important—read first:

Do not move the person or let him move unless his life is threatened by an immediate danger.

Do not twist or bend the injured person's back, neck, or head.

To prevent shock, cover the person lightly to keep him warm, but do not change his position.

Seek medical assistance immediately.

The most important step in first aid for a known or suspected back or neck injury is immobilization of the injured person to prevent spinal-cord damage.

If—and only if—the injured person is endangered by fire or another immediate threat to life, has no pulse, is not breathing, or is vomiting, follow instructions on these pages. If none of these dangers exists, follow instructions under **How to immobilize,** page 17.

Signs of back or neck injury

If an accident victim is conscious, question him for

☐ Pain in the back or neck
☐ Paralysis or weakness of an arm or leg
☐ Numbness or tingling of an arm or leg

Assume unconscious accident victims have back or neck injuries and treat as such.

Doctor's comments:
    Back and neck injuries commonly result from severe falls or automobile accidents. The spine is composed of small bones (vertebrae) that surround and protect the spinal cord. A broken vertebra may crush or cut the cord, causing paralysis, shock, or even death. This is why moving the injured person is to be avoided except when his life is threatened and why, when moving him, it is important not to bend or twist his neck or back.

Person face-down—4 rescuers

A1

A2

Person face-down—1 rescuer

A3

C To prevent choking, roll onto side

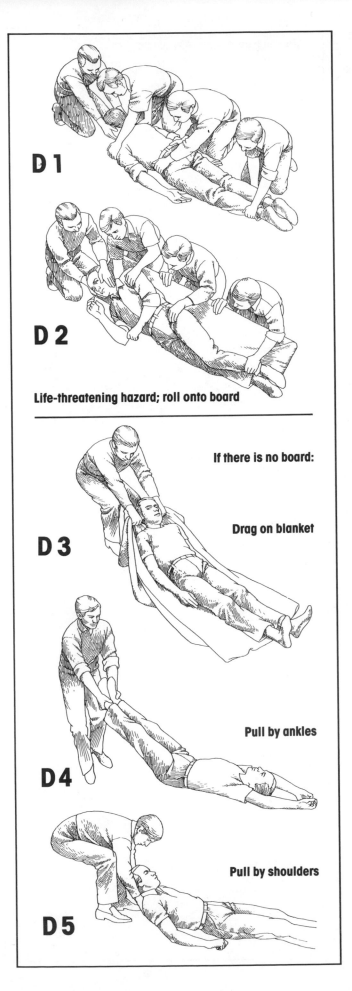

D 1

D 2

Life-threatening hazard; roll onto board

If there is no board:

Drag on blanket

D 3

Pull by ankles

D 4

Pull by shoulders

D 5

Move an accident victim only in the following life-threatening situations (if none exist, turn immediately to **How to immobilize** on the preceding page):

A. **The person is lying face-down** in a puddle, mud, etc., and cannot breathe. Roll him onto his back. Always roll the person as a single unit, never twisting or bending his back or neck.

1. Use four people, if possible: one holding the head and neck, one at the shoulders, one at the waist, one at the legs. If only two or three people are available, have one person hold the head and another hold the shoulders.

2. When the person holding the head says "go," roll all parts together, slowly and gently, keeping the head, neck, and torso in an unchanged alignment.
   OR

3. **If you are alone** with the injured person and are unable to summon help, stand behind his head, grasp his shoulders while steadying his head with your forearms, and drag him, still face-down, away from the puddle.

B. **The person has no pulse or is not breathing and needs CPR but is lying face-down.** Roll him onto his back as described above (A1&2). If you are alone, try to get help—roll him over by yourself only as a last resort, when CPR must be given immediately to restore breathing and pulse. Grasp him beneath the far arm and pull him toward you. Steady his head with your other hand to prevent twisting of his neck.

C. **The person is on his back and may choke** because of vomiting or bleeding in or around the mouth. Roll him onto his side, positioning people as described above (A1&2). Keep head, neck, and torso aligned, and provide support for the head. Do not roll the person by yourself. Seek assistance.

D. **The person's life is threatened by fire, explosion, or other danger** before medical help can arrive. Roll him onto his back on top of a long board, door, ironing board, etc., and bind him to it for emergency transportation.

1. Roll the person onto his side, positioning people as described above (A1&2), and place the board behind him.

2. Gently return board and person to the face-up position. Bind the person securely to the board, and carry board and person to safety.
   OR

3. If there is no board, roll the person onto a blanket and drag him to safety. Be sure his head and neck are held steady, and do not bend or twist him.

4. **If you are alone** with the injured person, or if there is no board, no blanket, or no time to use one, drag him to safety. Pull only in the direction in which his body is lying; never bend or twist him. On a smooth surface, pull by both ankles.
   OR

5. On a rough surface or a stairway, stand behind the person's head and pull him by the shoulders while steadying his head with your forearms.

After any of the above emergency procedures, the most important thing is to immobilize the person.

SEE INSTRUCTIONS ON THE PRECEDING PAGE.

Bites & Stings

overview:

First-aid principles for bites and stings include (1) limiting the spread of poisons through the body, (2) treating specific poisons, (3) controlling any bleeding, (4) observing shock and breathing difficulties, and treating them if necessary, (5) preventing infection by cleaning the bitten area, and (6) seeking medical care.

Specific treatment depends on what bit or stung you—see the appropriate section listed here. If you can't identify the source of a bite or sting, treat for the most severe possibility and seek medical attention immediately.

22-23 Snakebites First aid for poisonous and nonpoisonous bites

24 Snake identification guide A guide to poisonous and nonpoisonous snakes

25 Animal & human bites How to treat any wound caused by contact with the teeth of a warm-blooded animal

26-27 Spiders, scorpions & bees What to do for serious and potentially serious bites or stings. With identification guides

28-29 Ticks, chiggers, mosquitoes & other insects What to do for serious and minor bites and stings. With identification guides

30-31 Marine-life stings— cone shells, sea urchins, any stinging fish (except stingrays), and any unidentified marine life First aid for stings by these creatures, with identification guide—and for when you don't know what stung you

32-33 Marine-life stings—jellyfish, Portuguese men-of-war, stingrays, fire corals, sea anemones, hydras Different first-aid procedures for stings by each of these creatures. With identification guides

Bites & Stings
Snakebites

Important—read first:

Have someone else carefully **identify the snake** or kill it for identification at the hospital. **If you are the only rescuer, do this yourself if you can accomplish it quickly** before starting first aid. If **you** are bitten, don't exert yourself trying to kill the snake.

If you are unsure whether or not a snake is poisonous, assume that it is—play it safe.

Keep the bitten part immobile and below the level of the person's heart.

Do not give stimulants or alcoholic beverages or any pain medications before consulting a doctor.

After giving first aid, **treat for shock** by laying the person down and covering him with a blanket to keep him warm, unless you are sure that the snake is not poisonous. Watch carefully for breathing difficulties.

Calm the person as much as possible. Keep him from moving around. If he **must** walk to reach transportation, he should do so slowly.

Seek medical attention immediately for all possibly poisonous snakebites. Have someone phone ahead to alert the hospital, identifying the type of snake if possible (or take the dead snake with you). See a doctor for nonpoisonous snakebites as well.

People rarely die from snakebites, but pain and illness can be severe. To limit them, follow these steps **carefully but rapidly.**

Identify the type of snake if at all possible (see snake identification guide on next page). **If you are sure that it is not poisonous** (a pet snake, for instance), **wash the bitten area thoroughly with soap and water, and seek medical care.**

If the bite may be poisonous, start first aid with Step 1, preferably while someone else drives you and the victim to the nearest emergency room. **With coral-snake bites,** omit Steps 5 and 6 (cutting and suctioning the bite).

Doctor's comments:

Snakebites are rarely fatal, and recovery is ensured in almost all cases if medical care is received within an hour or two. But pain and illness can be severe, and damage to a bitten hand or foot can be disabling. You can decrease the severity of a snakebite by acting on three principles:

1. Rapid treatment with the correct antivenin is essential. Identifying the snake and phoning the hospital at once permits preparation of the appropriate serum. Transport the bitten person during or immediately after first aid has been administered, carrying and driving him so that he walks as little as possible.

2. Reducing the amount of venom in the wound and its spread to the rest of the body is just as important. This means thoroughly washing the bitten area, placing a band above it to close off veins (but not arteries), cutting and suctioning all but coral-snake bites (this should be attempted before reaching an emergency room **only** if you have the proper equipment and training and if you are more than one hour from medical assistance), keeping the bitten part low and immobilized, and slowing the person's circulation by not allowing him either to exercise or take stimulants, and providing him with reassurance.

3. Shock and respiratory failure—the most severe conditions that can follow snakebites—must be prevented or corrected.

There are four types of poisonous snakes in North America. Rattlesnakes, copperheads, and cottonmouths are called pit vipers because of the pit on each side of their heads, between eye and nostril. Their long fangs usually make distinctive marks but enter at an angle, so that shallow cuts are sufficient in drawing out their venom, which attacks the circulatory system.

Coral snakes, related to cobras, have short fangs. Their venom, which affects the nervous system, is spread over a wider area by chewing. This makes cutting and suction ineffective, and thorough washing essential.

Seek medical care even after nonpoisonous snakebites, because a tetanus shot or other treatment may be necessary.

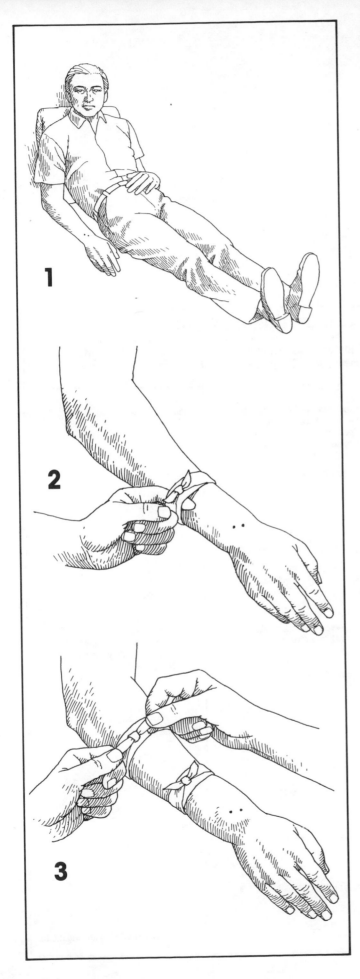

First aid for snakebites:

1. Have the person lie still, with the bitten part immobile and lower than his heart.

2. Tie a flat strip of cloth, a belt, or a watchband around a bitten arm or leg (**not** the head, neck, or torso) 2 to 4 inches above the bite. If a joint is in the way, place the strip above it. The strip should be snug but loose enough so that blood can ooze from the bite and there will be a pulse farther out on the limb. (A finger should be able to fit underneath the strip.) Check periodically, and loosen if necessary—but **do not remove.**

3. If swelling reaches the band, tie another band 2 to 4 inches higher up, then remove the first one.

4. Wash the bitten area thoroughly with soap and water. Flush it repeatedly if a coral-snake bite is suspected.

For all poisonous snakes EXCEPT CORAL SNAKES:

5. **Cutting.** Incising (cutting) a snakebite is controversial. If you are trained and have the appropriate equipment and are far from medical help, then you can incise a snake bite.

6. **Treat for shock** and be prepared to give artificial respiration if breathing stops, if you are trained in CPR.

7. **Seek medical attention immediately.** Have someone phone ahead to alert the hospital, identifying the type of snake if possible (or take the dead snake with you).

Bites & Stings
Identifying the snake

Important—read first:

There are two clues to the type of snake and its poisonous or nonpoisonous nature:

1. the snake's appearance
2. the type of bite marks

North American Snakes—Identification Guide

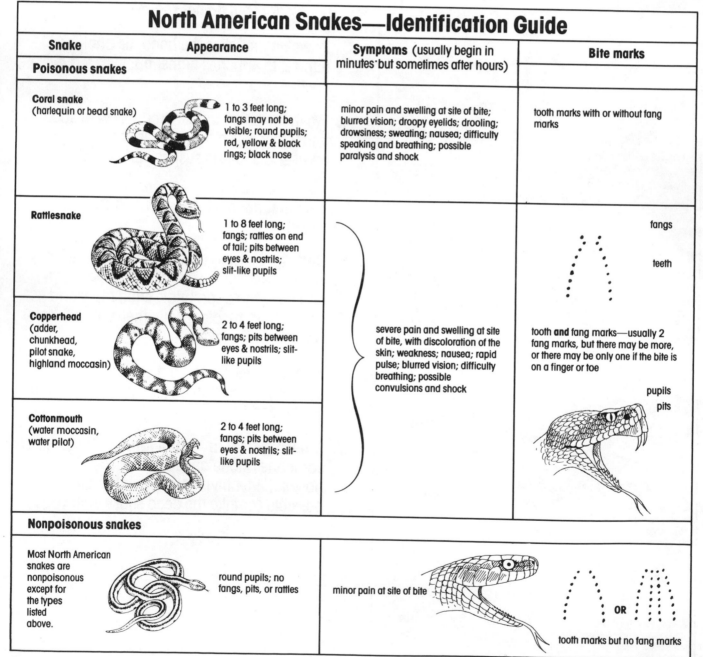

Snake	Appearance	Symptoms (usually begin in minutes but sometimes after hours)	Bite marks
Poisonous snakes			
Coral snake (harlequin or bead snake)	1 to 3 feet long; fangs may not be visible; round pupils; red, yellow & black rings; black nose	minor pain and swelling at site of bite; blurred vision; droopy eyelids; drooling; drowsiness; sweating; nausea; difficulty speaking and breathing; possible paralysis and shock	tooth marks with or without fang marks
Rattlesnake	1 to 8 feet long; fangs; rattles on end of tail; pits between eyes & nostrils; slit-like pupils	severe pain and swelling at site of bite, with discoloration of the skin; weakness; nausea; rapid pulse; blurred vision; difficulty breathing; possible convulsions and shock	fangs / teeth — tooth **and** fang marks—usually 2 fang marks, but there may be more, or there may be only one if the bite is on a finger or toe — pupils / pits
Copperhead (adder, chunkhead, pilot snake, highland moccasin)	2 to 4 feet long; fangs; pits between eyes & nostrils; slit-like pupils		
Cottonmouth (water moccasin, water pilot)	2 to 4 feet long; fangs; pits between eyes & nostrils; slit-like pupils		
Nonpoisonous snakes			
Most North American snakes are nonpoisonous except for the types listed above.	round pupils; no fangs, pits, or rattles	minor pain at site of bite	tooth marks but no fang marks OR

Bites & Stings
Animal & human bites

Important—read first:

Control any serious bleeding before giving other first aid (see **Bleeding,** page 35).

Get the name and address of the owner of a domestic animal that has bitten the victim. Carefully capture a wild animal that has bitten; kill it if you have to.

Do not give medicine or put any ointment, spray, medication, or household remedy on the bite until you've consulted a doctor.

Seek medical attention for **all** human and animal bites.

Any time human or animal teeth break skin, consider the wound to be a bite. The same bacteria get into a wound whether a hand hits teeth or teeth bite a hand.

If the bite has caused serious bleeding, control it first.

Then, quickly get the address of the animal's owner or capture the animal so that it can be checked for rabies. If you must kill it, try not to damage its head.

When these urgent steps are completed, follow first-aid directions

1. Wash the bite **thoroughly** with soap and water to remove saliva and other contamination. Continue washing for 5 full minutes.

2. **Control any minor bleeding** by covering the entire wound with a thick sterile gauze or clean cloth pad; if necessary, use your bare hand after washing it first. Press firmly on the entire wound. Put some ice against the pad—not directly on the skin.

3. While you press, raise the injury above the level of the heart.

4. When the bleeding has stopped, cover the bite with a sterile bandage or clean cloth tied or taped in place.

5. If the bandage is on an arm or leg, feel for a pulse farther out on the limb. If there is no pulse, loosen the bandage a bit.

Doctor's comments:

Bites by humans and animals, especially cats, are dangerous chiefly because of infections that result from bacteria in the mouth. Cleansing should be very thorough.

Any bite can cause tetanus. A tetanus booster shot is necessary if none has been received in five to eight years.

Rabies is a special danger in bites. Once the disease produces symptoms, it is nearly always fatal, but modern treatment can totally prevent rabies. The newest rabies vaccine is effective, safe, less painful, and requires fewer shots.

Rabies may be carried by all warm-blooded animals, especially dogs, bats, skunks, raccoons, foxes, rats, and squirrels. Although a rabid animal may not appear ill in the early stages of the disease, it can spread rabies by biting or even by licking a person's existing wound or sore. Rabies treatment for a bitten person may be safely delayed as long as the animal shows no symptoms—provided the bite was not too severe or too close to the head. Animals may be either confined and observed or killed so that their brains can be tested for rabies. Check with your local health department about the presence of rabies in your area. As a general rule, unprovoked attacks are more worrisome. Report all animal bites to the Board of Health or the police department.

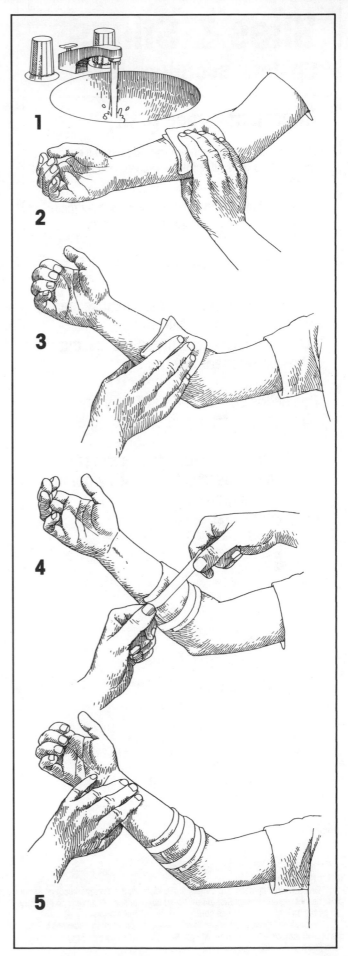

Bites & Stings
Spiders, scorpions & bees

Important—read first:

Observe for shock and be prepared to treat it after giving first aid for all spider, scorpion, and bee stings.

Seek medical attention for all spider and scorpion bites, for multiple bee stings, and for allergic reactions to bees.

Black widow spider, brown recluse spider, scorpion, and tarantula bites are serious and require immediate first aid followed by medical care.

Bee stings can be serious if they are numerous or if the person is allergic to them.

Identify the source of a bite or sting from the pictures, descriptions, and symptoms given in the guides, then follow the appropriate first-aid instructions.

Serious bites & stings: spiders & scorpions

Name	Appearance	Symptoms
Black widow spider	brown or black, with red or yellow hourglass on belly of female (male is not poisonous)	immediate redness and sharp pain; sweating; nausea; stomach and muscle cramps; difficult breathing; possible convulsions
Brown recluse (violin) spider	yellow or tan, with dark violin-shaped mark on back	delayed (2-8 hours) pain; swelling and blisters; rash; nausea; fever; joint pain; possible ulcer at site of bite
Tarantula	large spider with hairy body and legs	usually only slight local pain; occasionally produces reactions like black widow spider (above) or ulcer at site of bite
Scorpion	like a little lobster with a set of pincers at the end of its tail	burning pain, numbness or tingling; nausea; fever; stomach cramps; difficulty speaking; possible convulsions and shock

Potentially serious stings: bees

Bee	Appearance	Symptoms
Honey bee	hairy yellow or white and black body	local swelling, pain, redness, itching & burning at the site of the sting.
Hornet	not hairy; narrower or pinched waist; brown, black, red or striped body.	**Multiple stings:** headache; fever; muscle cramps; drowsiness; possible unconsciousness.
Yellow jacket		**Allergic reaction:** swelling elsewhere on the body, especially the face; weakness; wheezing; coughing; nausea; stomach cramps; blue skin; dizziness; possible unconsciousness.
Wasp		

Doctor's comments:

Black widow spiders, brown recluse spiders, and scorpions inject powerful poisons that require prompt first aid and medical attention. Tarantulas do this only rarely, but their bites often cause considerable localized damage.

All bees and wasps can cause severe, even life-threatening, reactions in allergic individuals, or with numerous stings. Be on the safe side by taking the precautions listed and watching closely for reactions.

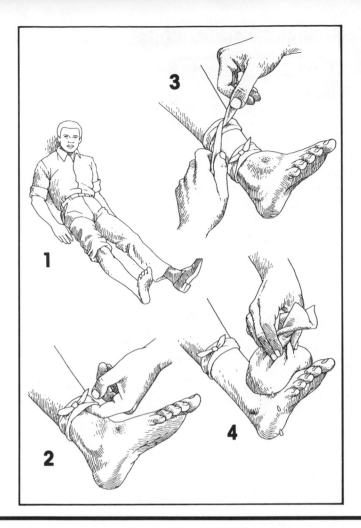

First aid for
spider and scorpion bites:

1. Have the person lie still, with the bitten part immobile and lower than his heart.

2. Tie a flat strip of cloth, a belt, or a watchband around a bitten arm or leg (not the head, neck, or torso) 2 to 4 inches above the bite. If a joint is in the way, place the strip above it. The strip should be snug but loose enough to allow a pulse farther out on the limb. (A finger should be able to fit underneath the strip.) Check periodically and loosen if necessary.

3. If swelling reaches the band, tie another band 2 to 4 inches higher up, then remove the first one. After 30 minutes, remove the constricting band.

4. Apply ice wrapped in cloth or a cold compress to the bite. Do not apply ice directly to the skin.

5. Observe for signs of shock or difficulty breathing.

6. Seek medical attention immediately.

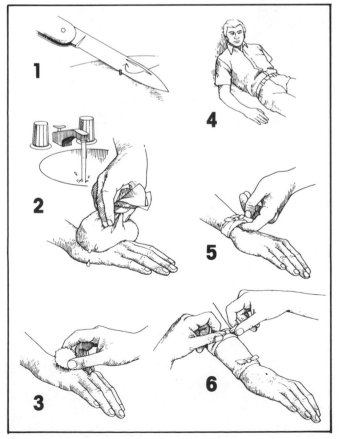

First aid for bee stings:

1. Only a honey bee leaves its stinger in the skin. Only if it is visible, carefully remove it with the edge of a razor, a knife, or a fingernail. Do not squeeze the stinger, as this will inject more venom.

2. Wash all bee stings with soap and water. If the person is allergic to bee stings, put ice wrapped in cloth or a cold compress on the sting to decrease pain and the absorption of venom. Do not put ice directly on the skin.

3. Relieve pain with calamine lotion or a baking soda and water paste.

   If you know that the person is allergic to bee stings, seek medical attention immediately (after removing a honey bee stinger). If symptoms appear suggesting the beginning of an allergic reaction or a reaction to multiple stings, and the stings are on the arm or leg:

4. Have the person lie still with the stung part immobile and lower than his heart.

5. Tie a flat strip of cloth, a belt, or a watchband around the arm or leg (not the head, neck, or torso) 2 to 4 inches above the sting. If a joint is in the way, place the strip above it. The strip should be snug but loose enough to allow a pulse farther out on the limb. (A finger should be able to fit underneath the strip.) Check periodically and loosen if necessary—but do not remove it.

6. If swelling reaches the band, tie another band 2 to 4 inches higher up, then remove the first one.

7. Seek medical attention immediately.

Bites & Stings
Ticks, chiggers, mosquitoes & other insects

Important—read first:

Seek medical attention for fever or infection following a tick or mosquito bite.

Ticks must be properly and promptly removed to prevent possible disease. Mosquito and other insect bites are rarely serious but may require care to relieve discomfort.

Identify the source of a bite from the guides, if possible; then follow the appropriate first-aid instructions.

First aid for tick bites:

1. Remove the tick with your fingers if it is not holding onto the skin. Crush it.

2. If the tick will not come off easily, **do not pull.** Make the tick let go by covering it with Vaseline, thick oil, gasoline, or kerosene (beware of fire). Then pull it off carefully and completely with tweezers.

3. Wash the bite thoroughly with soap and water.

4. **Seek medical attention if the bite becomes infected.** Signs of infection may appear in hours or days. They include tenderness, throbbing, pus, redness, and swelling around the bite; red streaks leading from it; swollen glands; and fever. Also seek medical care for any fever occurring within 10 days of a tick bite, regardless of other symptoms.

Doctor's comments:
Ticks are notorious for their ability to burrow into the skin and hang on. Pulling on an embedded tick may remove the body, leaving the head in the skin to cause infection. Prompt and complete removal is essential for two reasons: (1) On rare occasions, ticks cause temporary paralysis, which stops as soon as they are removed. (2) In many parts of the country, ticks can carry Rocky Mountain Spotted Fever and other illnesses. They rarely transmit these diseases if removed within an hour.

The bites of other insects are rarely more than annoying, but a number of serious diseases can be transmitted, especially by mosquitoes. Mosquito-borne illnesses usually begin with fever. In the tropics, these include malaria and yellow fever. In the United States, especially in the South and Southwest, mosquitoes can transmit encephalitis.

Potentially serious bites: ticks

Creature	Appearance	Symptoms
ticks are found in trees and shrubs and on animals	very tiny oval body; gray or brown	usually none; local infection if incompletely removed; rarely, paralysis until removed; occasionally, fever days later

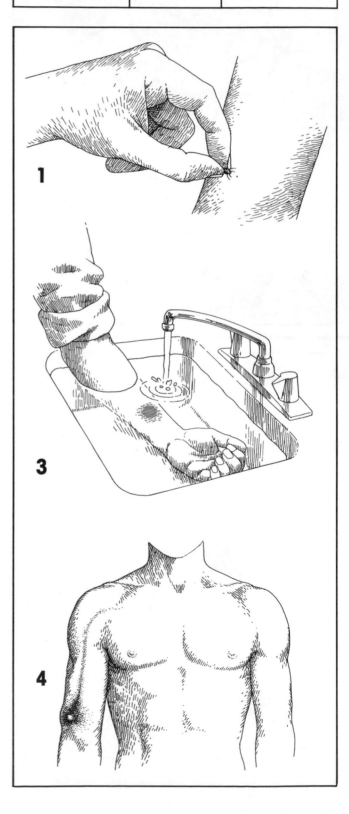

Minor bites and stings: insects

Insect (and where found)	Appearance	Symptoms
Bedbug (in crevices, under wallpaper)	yellow, red or brown; flat, oval body; 6 legs	burning or stinging sensation at the site of the bite; redness, swelling and itching
Chigger (in damp vegetation)	red or colorless; 6 or 8 legs; velvety hair on body	
Flea (on animals)	6 long legs; jumps extremely well	
Gnat (everywhere)	tiny, dark insect which may be barely visible	
Mosquito (everywhere)	thin, dark body; transparent wings; long mouth parts	

First aid for minor bites and stings:

1. Wash the affected area thoroughly with soap and water.

2. Relieve itching with cold, wet compresses, calamine lotion, or a paste made of baking soda and a little water.

3. **Seek medical attention** if scratching leads to a secondary infection. Signs of infection, which may appear in hours or days, include tenderness, throbbing, pus, redness and swelling around the bite; red streaks leading from it; swollen glands and fever.

4. **Seek medical attention for any fever beginning within 10 days of an insect bite.** Mosquitoes, fleas and bedbugs, and less common insects which may resemble them, can transmit a variety of illnesses (usually with fever) in certain geographic areas.

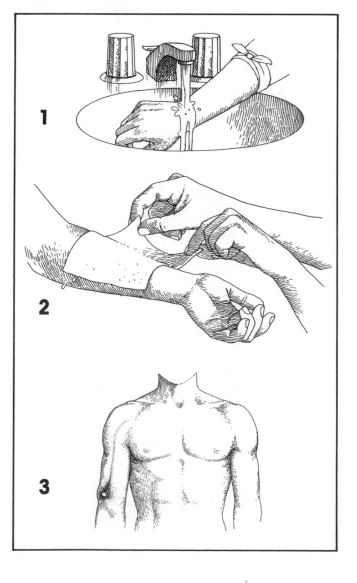

Bites & Stings

Marine-life stings— cone shells, sea urchins, any stinging fish (except stingrays) & any unidentified marine life

Important—read first:

Control any serious bleeding before giving other first aid (see **Bleeding,** page 35).

Observe for shock and difficulty in breathing, and, if you are properly trained, be prepared to treat these conditions after giving first aid for any marine-life sting.

Seek medical attention immediately for all marine-life stings.

Marine-life stings can be extremely painful but rarely result in permanent damage or death. A number of marine animals can produce poisonous stings when brushed against or stepped on. The most common and easily identified are pictured and described in this and the following section.

Swimmers are occasionally stung by saltwater and freshwater fish such as catfish, dogfish, weaverfish, scorpion fish, and eels. Often the source of an underwater sting is not known. In these cases, follow the instructions on the opposite page.

Cone shells & sea urchins

Creature	Appearance	Symptoms
Cone shell	1 to 3 inches long; cone-shaped shell, with wavy stripes or an irregular pattern	pain; swelling; numbness or tingling; dizziness; blurred vision; difficulty breathing and swallowing; possible paralysis and collapse
Sea urchin	rounded; size of a golf ball or tennis ball; sharp spines	pain; swelling; dizziness; muscle weakness and possible paralysis

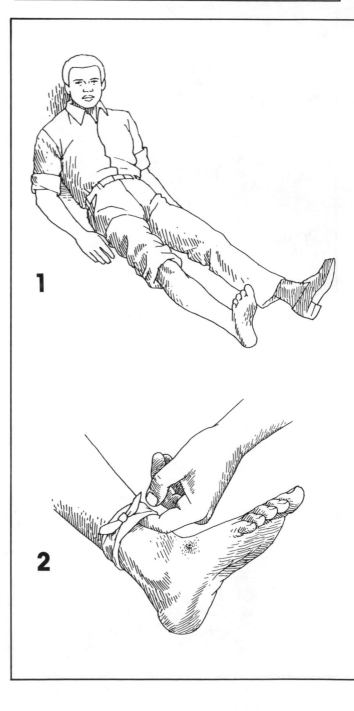

1

2

Doctor's comments:
There are no effective antidotes for the stings of cone shells, sea urchins or most fish. First aid focuses on reducing the amount of venom in the wound and its spread to the rest of the body. This means washing the sting thoroughly, removing loose material and stingers, using a band to close off veins (but not arteries) and having the person lie still with the stung part lower than his heart.

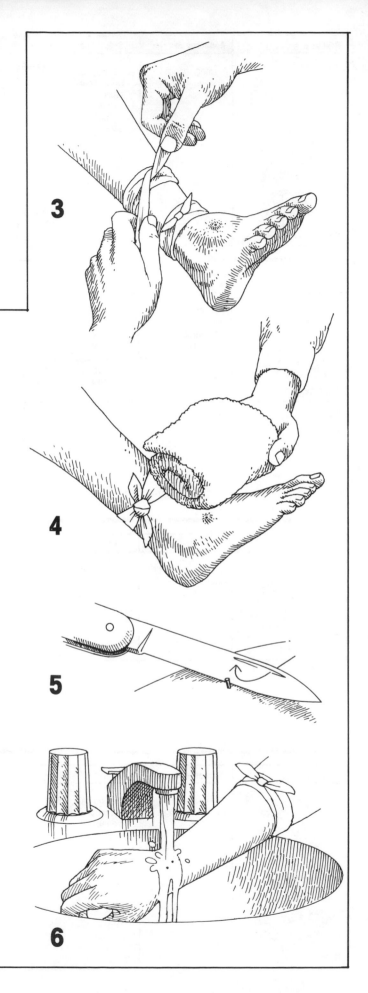

First aid for stings from cone shells, sea urchins, any stinging fish (except stingrays), and any unidentified marine life:

1. Have the person lie still, with the stung part immobile and lower than his heart.

2. Tie a flat strip of cloth, a belt, or a watchband around a stung arm or leg (**not** the head, neck, or torso) 2 to 4 inches above the sting. If a joint is in the way, place the strip above it. The strip should be snug but loose enough to allow a pulse farther out on the limb. (A finger should be able to fit underneath the strip.) Check periodically; and loosen if necessary—but **do not remove it.**

3. If swelling reaches the band, tie another band 2 to 4 inches higher up, then remove the first one.

4. Use a towel or tweezers to remove any loose material at the site of the sting.

5. Remove any stingers with the edge of a knife or razor. Move the blade upward from the skin to lift them out. **Do not squeeze the stingers,** as this will inject more venom.

6. Wash the site of the sting thoroughly with soap and water.

7. Observe carefully for signs of shock or breathing difficulty.

8. **Seek medical attention.**

Bites & Stings

Marine-life stings—jellyfish, Portuguese men-of-war, stingrays, fire corals, sea anemones & hydras

Important—read first:

Control any serious bleeding before giving other first aid (see **Bleeding,** page 35).

Observe for shock and difficulty in breathing, and, if you are properly trained, be prepared to treat these conditions after giving first aid for any marine-life sting.

Seek medical attention immediately for all marine-life stings.

Marine-life stings can be extremely painful but rarely result in permanent damage or death.

It is important (and easy) to identify the creatures in this section, because the treatment for each type of sting is different.

Creature	Appearance	Symptoms
Jellyfish / Portuguese man-of-war	floating sacs or discs with trailing tentacles	burning pain; red skin and rash; muscle cramps; nausea; possible difficulty breathing; possible shock

Creature	Appearance	Symptoms
Stingray	flat, shark-like fish with rough skin and barbed, whip-like tail	severe pain; area of sting turns pale, then red; sweating; dizziness; nausea; weakness; possible paralysis and collapse

Creature	Appearance	Symptoms
Fire coral (stinging coral)	rounded clusters of short branches; color varies	burning pain

Creature	Appearance	Symptoms
Sea anemone / Hydra	flower-like; immobile; long tentacles	burning pain; chills; stomach cramps; diarrhea

Doctor's comments:
There are specific antidotes for all the marine-life stings in this section except fire coral. Alcohol or ammonia neutralizes jellyfish and man-of-war toxins. The poisons injected by stingrays, sea anemones, and hydras are inactivated by heat.

Stingray wounds and fire coral scrapes often result in bleeding. While this helps remove the toxins that have been injected, it may be severe enough to require direct pressure on the wound to control blood loss. Other stings can occur when someone slips on rocks or coral; cuts and bleeding, unrelated to the sting itself, may also require first aid.

First aid for jellyfish and Portuguese man-of-war stings:

1. Wrap your hand in a towel or cloth and wipe away all attached tentacles.

2. Wash the area with alcohol or ammonia and saltwater (**do not** use freshwater).

3. Observe carefully for signs of shock or breathing difficulty.

4. **Seek medical attention.**

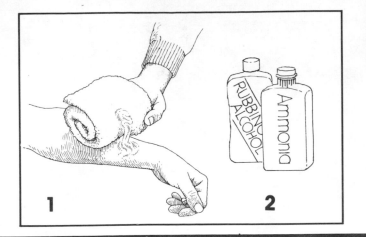

First aid for stingray stings:

1. Remove all loose material from the area of the wound with a towel or tweezers. An embedded bony spine will probably require surgical removal.

2. Soak the area in water that is as hot as possible without scalding the person. Continue for 30 minutes to 1 hour, using hot soaks while on the way to the doctor.

3. Treat for shock. Lay the person down and cover him with a blanket to keep him warm.

4. Check breathing, and be prepared to give artificial respiration, if you are trained in CPR.

5. **Seek medical attention immediately.**

First aid for fire coral (stinging coral) stings:

1. Wash the wound thoroughly with soap and water.

2. Observe carefully for signs of shock or breathing difficulty.

3. **Seek medical attention.**

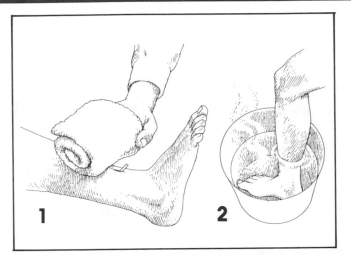

First aid for sea anemone and hydra stings:

1. Soak the stung area in water that is as hot as possible without scalding the person. Continue for 30 minutes to 1 hour, using hot soaks while on the way to the doctor.

2. Observe carefully for signs of shock or breathing difficulty.

3. **Seek medical attention.**

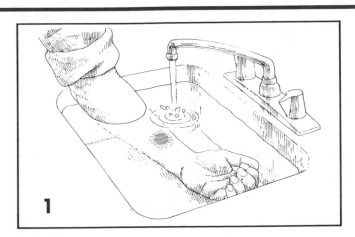

Bleeding

overview:

It is natural to react with fear to the sight of blood, but if you can remain calm, you can control bleeding with the techniques described in this chapter.

Bleeding may be apparent (external) or inapparent (internal). External bleeding is stopped by direct pressure. The signs of internal bleeding must be recognized, and require immediate medical assistance.

37 Direct pressure

38 Tourniquet

40 Amputation (loss of an ear lobe, finger, toe, or other body part)

42 Nosebleeds (spontaneous)

43 Internal bleeding

Bleeding
Direct pressure

Important—read first:

Do not remove impaled objects.

Do not remove bandages if they become blood-soaked; you may disturb the clot and cause bleeding to resume. Just add another layer on top and press harder.

Seek medical attention.

1. Cover the entire wound with a thick sterile or clean cloth pad. Gauze, clean towels, undershirts, and pieces of a sheet make excellent pads. Use ice or cold water in the pad to help stop bleeding and decrease swelling. If no clean cloth is available, use your bare hands—wash them first if possible.

2. Press firmly on the entire wound for ten minutes without releasing pressure.

3. While you press, raise the injury above the level of the person's heart. You may need to change his position.

4. When the bleeding stops, secure the pad firmly. If the bandage is on a limb, periodically feel for a pulse farther out on the limb. If there is no pulse, loosen the bandage a bit.

5. **If bleeding has not stopped, you are not pressing hard enough, press harder.**

6. If bleeding still cannot be stopped and bleeding is from a limb, use a tourniquet (see next page).

7. Seek medical attention.

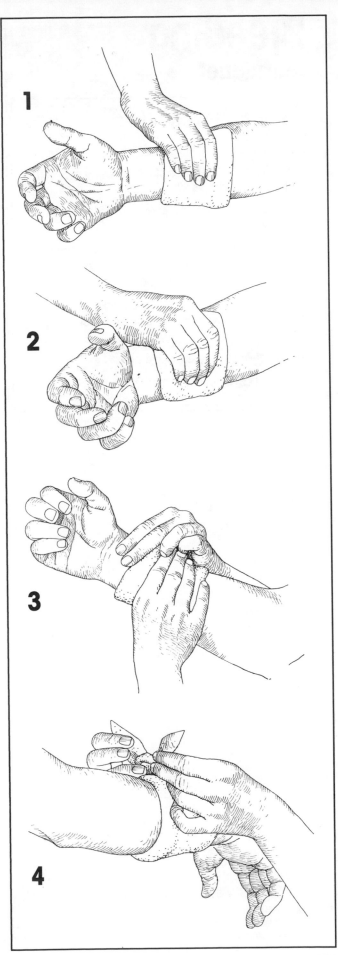

Doctor's comments:
Seek medical attention if the bleeding was caused by a serious injury or if stitches are needed to keep the wound closed. An open wound is prone to infection. See a doctor if a tetanus booster has not been received within the last 10 years.

Bleeding
Tourniquet

Important—read first:

Do not remove impaled objects.

Use a tourniquet only in a life-threatening situation and only as a last resort.

Use a tourniquet only on an arm or leg, never on the head, neck, or torso.

A tourniquet can damage nerves and other tissues with its heavy, direct pressure. For this reason, it is safest to use a wide, flat cloth strip.

Do not remove a tourniquet once it has been applied. More severe bleeding could occur.

Do not cover a tourniquet. It must be seen immediately by medical personnel.

Seek medical attention immediately.

1

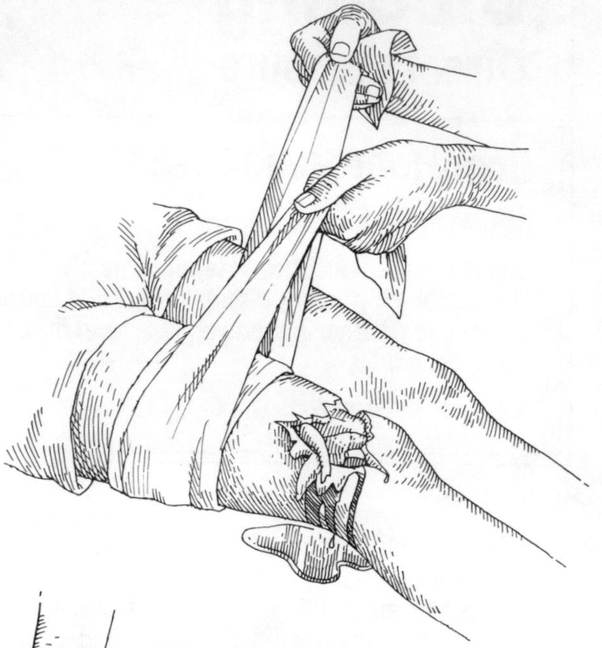

2

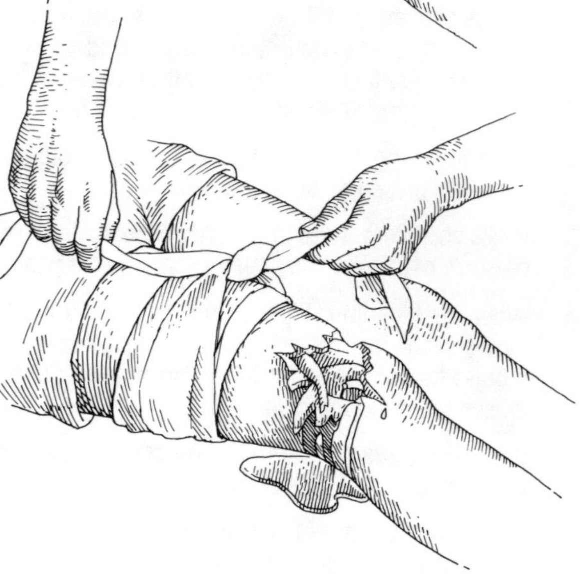

3

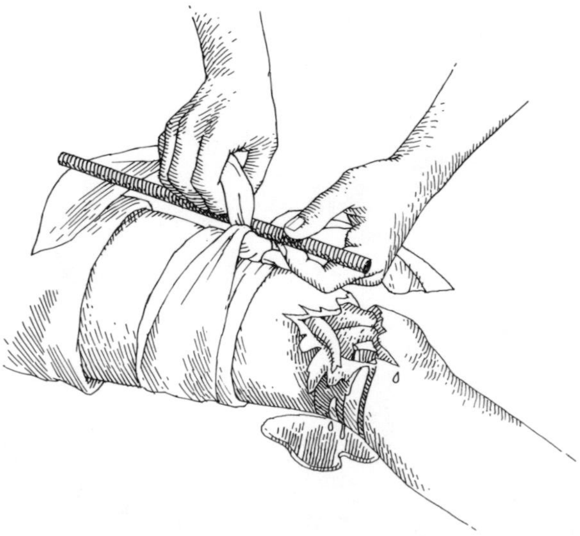

Doctor's comments:
A tourniquet will stop even the most severe bleeding from an arm or leg, but it may cause damage—even loss of the limb—because it cuts off the flow of blood so thoroughly.

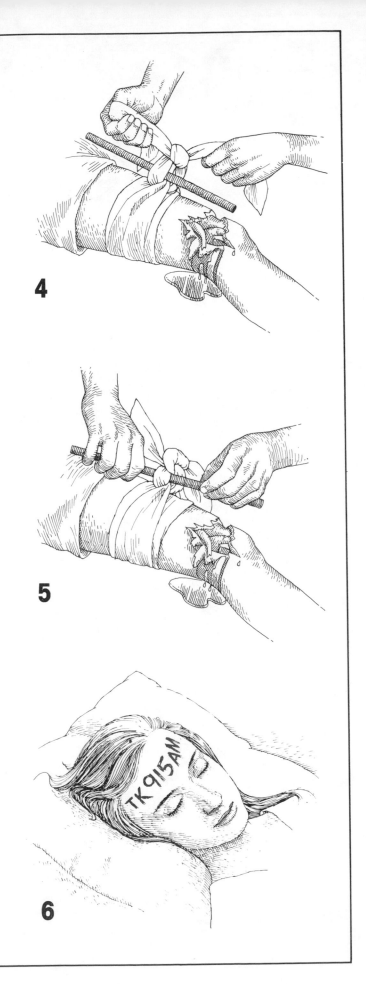

Applying a tourniquet if severe bleeding can't be stopped

1. Find a cloth at least 2 inches wide (a scarf, a wide piece of sheet, a piece of clothing, etc.). Never use a thin strip of cloth, a belt, a cord, or wire as a tourniquet. The cloth must be long enough to go around the limb 3 times. Place your tourniquet above the wound but not touching it. If a joint or a fracture is in the way, place the tourniquet above it. Keeping the cloth flat and tight, wrap it twice around the limb.

2. Tie a half-knot with the ends of the cloth.

3. Place a strong, fairly straight stick on top of the knot. You can use an eating utensil, a tent peg, a large pen, etc., between 5 and 10 inches long.

4. Then tie a double knot over the stick.

5. Twist the stick until the bleeding stops, but no tighter. Tie the stick securely in place with the loose ends of the tourniquet or with a second cloth strip.

6. On a scrap of paper or cloth, write "tourniquet" and the time it was applied; attach this to the person's clothing. Or use lipstick to write "TK" and the time on the person's forehead.

7. Do not remove or cover the tourniquet.

Bleeding
Amputation
(loss of an earlobe, finger, toe, or other body part)

Important—read first:

Stop bleeding by applying direct pressure to the wound.

Seek medical attention immediately. Notify the hospital, if possible, that an amputation victim is on the way.

If time permits, look for and save the severed part, wrap it in a cold, damp cloth, and make sure that it accompanies the person to the hospital.

The first step in controlling bleeding is to apply direct pressure to the wound.

If direct pressure does not stop severe bleeding, see **Bleeding: Tourniquet** (previous page).

After you have controlled bleeding, care for the amputated part.

Follow instructions at right.

Doctor's comments:

    Many amputations (for example, of fingers, toes, parts of the ear) do not involve severe bleeding. Even a major amputation may not cause massive bleeding, since the ends of blood vessels often constrict, and the control of bleeding can frequently be accomplished without the use of a tourniquet.

    Reattachment of severed limbs is often possible today, especially if the hospital has been alerted and can prepare its staff and equipment. Try to keep the severed part moist, cool (to reduce its need for oxygen), and clean. If possible, wrap the severed part in a damp cloth, put it in a plastic bag, and place it in a container filled with ice.

    While care for the amputated part is important, it is never as important as continued care for the injured person.

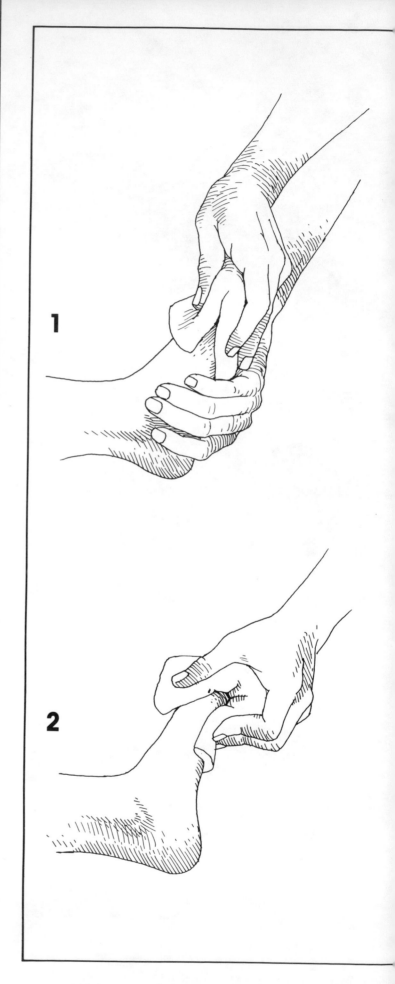

1

2

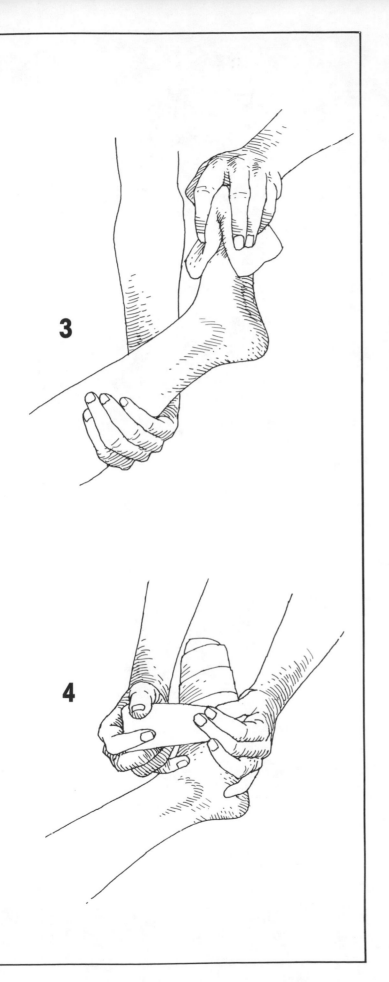

Direct pressure

1. First, cover the entire wound with a thick, clean cloth pad. Use gauze, a towel, clothing, or your bare hands if necessary.

2. Then press firmly on the entire wound.

3. As you press, raise the wound above the level of the person's heart.

4. When the bleeding stops, secure the pad firmly.

Tourniquet

5. Use a tourniquet only if absolutely necessary to stop life-threatening bleeding. Use only on an arm or leg. For complete instructions, see page 38.

Care for the amputated part

6. Wrap the part in a cold, damp cloth, but do not put it in water.

7. Place the wrapped part in a plastic bag, if possible, and put the closed bag inside a second container full of ice. Avoid direct contact between the part and the ice.

Bleeding
Nosebleeds (spontaneous)

Important—read first:

For a broken nose, see **Nose Injuries,** page 134.

Seek medical attention if severe bleeding persists for more than 15 minutes.

Giving calm reassurance is important in all cases of nosebleeds.

1. Have the person sit leaning slightly forward so that blood does not run down his throat. Have the person spit out any blood in his mouth, as swallowing it may cause gagging and vomiting.

2. Have the person pinch his nose firmly but gently for 10 full minutes, using his thumb and forefinger; then release slowly.

3. While the person is pinching, apply a cold compress to the nose and the surrounding area. (If you are doing the pinching yourself, ask a helper to get the compress.)

4. If pinching does not work, gently pack the nostril (both nostrils if you are unsure of the source of the blood). Use gauze or a clean strip of cloth (not absorbent cotton, which will stick). Use only one strip in each nostril, and be sure that both ends of the strip hang out, to facilitate removal later. Then pinch the nose, with the gauze in it, for another 5 minutes.

Doctor's comments:

Nosebleeds are usually minor. They are commonly caused by irritation due to colds, allergies, picking, or overuse of nose drops or sprays. On occasion, nosebleeds can be dangerously severe, particularly in adults with high blood pressure.

If a foreign object or large clots in the nose make pinching it painful or impossible, they can be gently blown out first. Do not attempt to remove a foreign object that cannot be gently blown free by the person; seek medical assistance.

After a nosebleed stops, do not irritate or blow the nose for several hours.

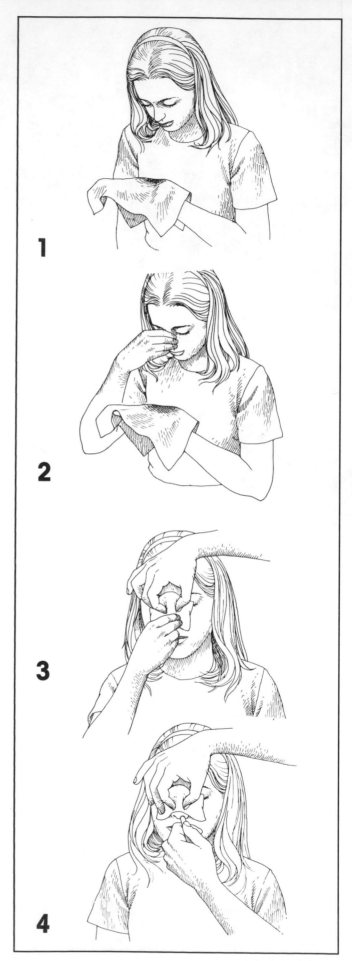

1

2

3

4

Bleeding
Internal bleeding

Important—read first:

Do not give the person anything to eat or drink, as surgery may be necessary.

Conserve body heat by covering the person lightly. A blanket should be placed underneath him if the ground is cold. But do not overheat the person.

Seek medical assistance immediately.

Suspect internal bleeding if any of the following signs appears after an injury:

- ☐ Coughing, with foamy, red blood
- ☐ Vomiting, with red or brown "coffee-ground" material
- ☐ Bowel movements containing red or black tar-like material
- ☐ Red or brown urine

A. If the person is unconscious, is vomiting, or is bleeding in or around the mouth, lay him on his side to keep his airway open.

B. In all other situations, have the person lie on his back with his legs elevated 8 to 12 inches. Seek medical assistance immediately.

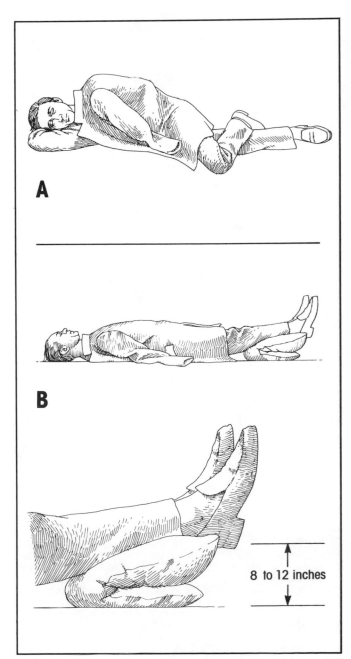

A

B

8 to 12 inches

Doctor's comments:
Suspected internal bleeding or bleeding from major wounds in the stomach area require immediate medical attention.

Breaks, Sprains
& Dislocations

overview:

Fractures (broken bones), sprains (stretched or torn joint ligaments), and dislocations (bone ends out of place) are rarely life-threatening, but they can lead to prolonged pain and disability if they are not treated promptly and properly.

The next page lists the signs of bone and joint injuries and explains the principles of treatment: (1) first treating any life-threatening condition, such as breathing difficulty, loss of pulse, and bleeding when the injury is the result of a serious accident and you are properly trained in CPR; (2) keeping movement of the person and the injured part to a minimum; (3) immobilizing the injured part with splints, slings, and bandages; (4) avoiding contamination of open bone injuries; (5) preventing swelling—especially when joints are involved; and (6) treating for shock if necessary.

Succeeding pages give step-by-step instructions for the use of splints, slings, and bandages to immobilize specific bones or joints.

46 **General principles for treating bone and joint injuries**

48-49 **Shoulder blade & collarbone**

50-51 **Upper arm**

52-53 **Elbow**

54-55 **Forearm, wrist, hand & fingers**

56-57 **Pelvis**

58-59 **Hip & upper leg**

60-61 **Knee**

62-63 **Lower leg**

64 **Ankle, foot & toes**

Breaks & Sprains
General principles for treating bone and joint injuries

Important—read first:

If a neck or back injury is suspected, do not move the person. Turn to **Back & Neck Injuries,** page 15, for instructions.

Signs of possible bone or joint injuries

Suspect a bone or joint injury after any accident when one or more of these signs appear:

☐ Pain or tenderness over a bone or joint
☐ The person heard or felt a "snap"
☐ Inability to move an injured limb
☐ Numbness, tingling, or loss of pulse in an injured limb
☐ A grating sound or feeling
☐ Swelling or bluish discoloration over a bone or joint
☐ Abnormal shape, position, or movement of a bone or joint

If an accident victim is unconscious, gently feel the entire body for possible bone injuries.

What to do for all possible bone or joint injuries (except of the back or neck)

Without x-rays, even doctors can't always tell fractures (broken bones), dislocations (bone ends out of place), and sprains (stretched or torn ligaments) apart. And two or all three can occur together. So first-aid procedures for all three are the same. The major procedure is to immobilize the injured part, but first:

1. Treat any life-threatening condition if you are trained in CPR

If any injury is severe, check the person's pulse and breathing before you do anything else. If you are properly trained in CPR, give artificial respiration if necessary; otherwise, call for medical assistance. Next, control any severe bleeding at the site of a bone injury or elsewhere on the body. Then stabilize the injured bone or joint. But remember:

2. Keep movement of the injured person to a minimum

Do not move the person before the injured part has been immobilized (unless there is an immediate threat, such as fire). This is to avoid additional damage from tearing of nerves and blood vessels, the creation of more pain, bleeding, and even shock. If the injury can't be completely stabilized before transporting the person to a doctor, call for professional help to come to the scene. With injuries of the pelvis, hip, and upper leg, transport by ambulance if at all possible.

3. Immobilize with splints, slings, and bandages

The major first-aid procedure is to stabilize the injured bone or joint without changing its position. Do not try to straighten an injured part, except where specifically instructed to do so. Splints, slings, and bandages must immobilize the joints at both ends of a suspected broken bone or the bones on both sides of a suspected sprain or dislocation. (Instructions for immobilizing specific body parts are given on the following pages.)

Splints: If a board is not available, use a branch, a rolled magazine or newspaper, a broom, a pillow, an umbrella, or a bat. As a last resort, you can use another part of the person's own body—for example, use his uninjured leg to stabilize his broken leg. Splints may be tied on with cloth strips, sleeves torn from shirts, neckties, belts, and similar objects. Tie splints on snugly but not too tightly. Check for a pulse farther out on a limb after you have finished applying the splint; loosen if too tight. Check repeatedly to be sure that swelling hasn't caused the bandage to become too tight, and ask whether numbness or tingling has set in.

4. Avoid contamination of broken skin

If the skin over an injured bone has been cut, you may be dealing with an open, or "compound," fracture—regardless of whether the skin was cut from inside by the sharp bone end or from outside by the striking object. Contamination of a compound fracture can lead to severe infection of the bone. Keep an open fracture clean by covering it with the cleanest available cloth. Never apply medicine or try to push the bone ends back in. Aside from these precautions, treat open fractures the same as closed, or "simple," fractures, sprains, and dislocations.

5. Prevent swelling

Swelling is especially severe in joint injuries. Elevate injured joints and apply ice, wrapped in a towel or cloth. For a known sprain, applying heat after 24 hours have passed occasionally makes an injury feel better.

6. Treat for shock

After a bone or joint injury has been immobilized, check for shock and treat it if necessary, if you are properly trained in CPR techniques.

STEP-BY-STEP INSTRUCTIONS FOR IMMOBILIZING SPECIFIC PARTS OF THE BODY ARE GIVEN ON THE FOLLOWING PAGES.

Breaks & Sprains
Shoulder blade & collarbone

Important—read first:

Before immobilizing the injured area, keep movement to an absolute minimum.

Do not try to straighten the injured part.

If the skin over a suspected fracture is broken, do not touch it. Cover it with the cleanest available cloth.

Check pulse at the wrist periodically and check for numb fingers to be sure that a bandage is not too tight.

Seek medical attention immediately.

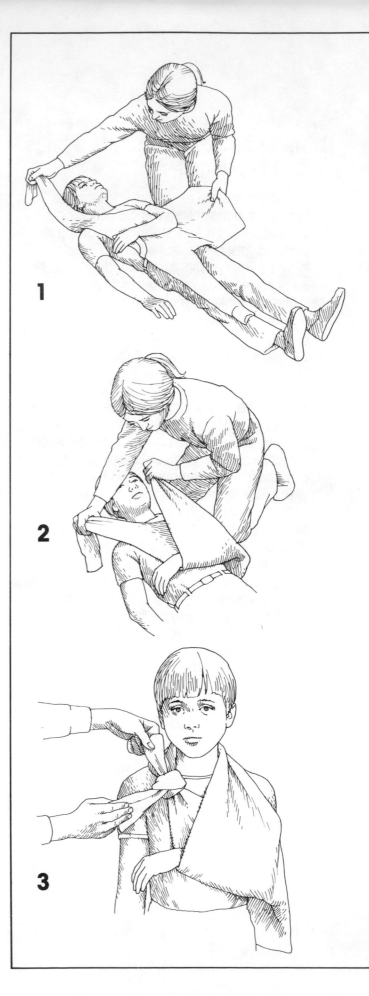

Doctor's comments:

A sling takes the weight of the arm off the injured shoulder blade or collarbone so that the person can sit or stand. A second bandage immobilizes the injured area by binding it to the person's chest.

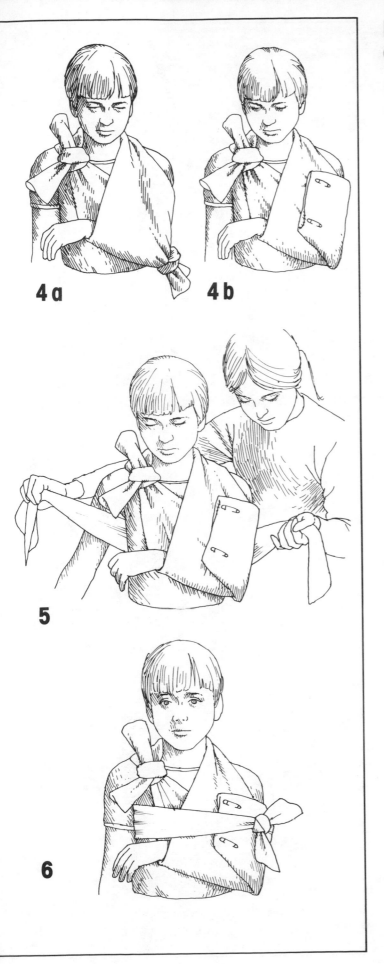

4 a   4 b

5

6

How to immobilize with a sling and second bandage

For any suspected injury to the shoulder blade or collarbone:

1. Place a large triangular bandage, or a shirt, on the person's chest, with one corner under the elbow on the injured side, one corner over the uninjured shoulder, and one corner down near the knees. Place the lower arm on the injured side across the person's chest at a right angle, with the hand about 4 inches higher than the elbow.

2. Bring the lowest corner of the bandage up over the injured shoulder.

3. Tie the two upper corners together. The knot should be on the side to avoid painful pressure on the neck.

4. Fold the third corner around the elbow on the injured side and (a) tie or (b) pin it in place. Be sure the fingers are not covered.

5. Pass a second long cloth strip around the person.

6. Wrap it around the person's chest, upper arm, and the sling, and tie it snugly. Check pulse at the wrist periodically and check for numb fingers; loosen bandages if necessary.

7. The person will probably be most comfortable sitting up while being transported to medical care.

Breaks & Sprains
Upper arm

Important—read first:

Before immobilizing the injured area, keep movement to an absolute minimum.

Do not try to straighten the injured upper arm bone.

If the skin over a suspected fracture is broken, do not touch it. Cover it with the cleanest available cloth.

Check pulse at the wrist periodically and check for numb fingers to be sure that a bandage is not too tight.

Seek medical attention immediately.

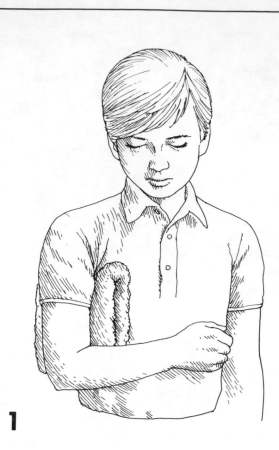

1

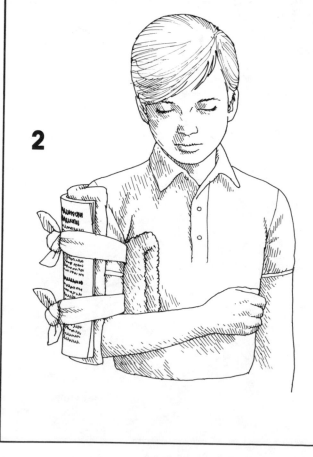

2

Doctor's comments:
This technique immobilizes the upper arm bone at three points. The splint immobilizes the broken bone ends. The narrow sling stabilizes the elbow without pressing on the upper arm bone. The final, wide bandage immobilizes the shoulder joint. The pad in the hollow under the arm keeps the broken bone aligned and absorbs perspiration.

How to immobilize with a splint, sling, and bandage

For any suspected injury to the bone between the shoulder and the elbow:

1. Place a pad about 1 inch thick (such as a folded face towel) in the person's armpit. Then place thé upper arm against the side of the chest, with the lower arm at a right angle across the chest.

2. Place a padded splint along the outer side of the upper arm. You can use a magazine, newspaper, or board with a small towel. Tie it to the arm above and below the suspected break.

3. Support the lower arm with a narrow sling (such as a necktie) around the neck and wrist. The knot should not press against the neck or the wrist.

4. Use a wide bandage, towel, etc., to bind the upper arm to the chest. This bandage goes over the splint and sling and under the other arm. Check pulse at the wrist periodically and check for numb fingers; loosen bandages if necessary.

5. The person will probably be most comfortable sitting up while being transported to medical care.

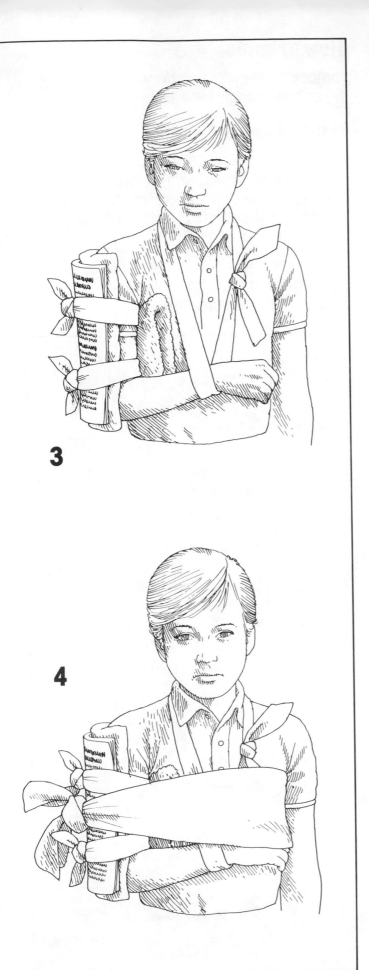

3

4

Breaks & Sprains
Elbow

Important—read first:

Before immobilizing the injured area, keep movement to an absolute minimum.

Do not try to bend or to straighten the elbow.

If the skin over a suspected fracture is broken, do not touch it. Cover it with the cleanest available cloth.

Check pulse at the wrist and check for numb fingers to be sure that a bandage is not too tight.

Seek medical attention immediately.

How to immobilize

Immobilize an injured elbow without changing its position or angle even slightly.

If the elbow is bent:

1. Support the elbow in the exact position in which it was found with a narrow sling (such as a necktie) around the neck and wrist The knot should not press against the neck or wrist.

2. Bind the upper arm to the chest with a wide bandage or towel going over the sling and under the other arm.

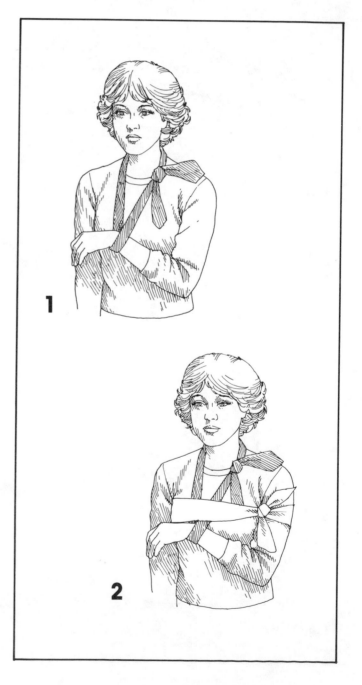

Doctor's comments:
Elbow injuries are very painful, and damage to arteries often causes internal bleeding and swelling of the joint. Ice and elevation during transportation or while waiting for help reduce the amount of swelling. Major nerves that lie next to the elbow joint may also be injured if the elbow is not carefully stabilized.

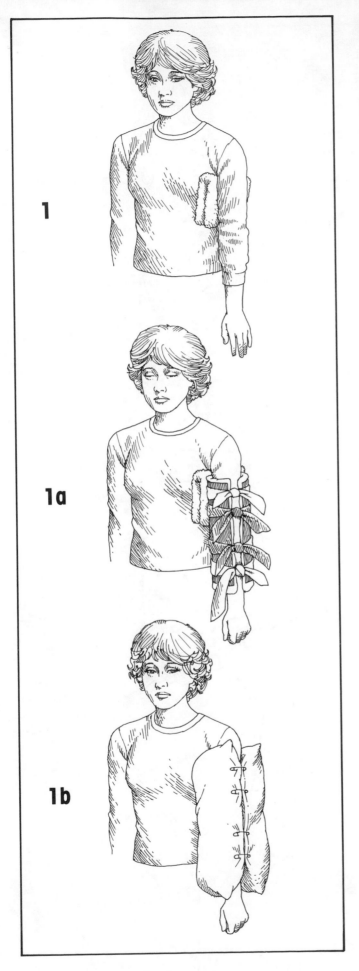

How to immobilize

Immobilize an injured elbow without changing its position or angle even slightly.

If the elbow is straight:

1. Place a pad about 1 inch thick (such as a folded face towel) in the person's armpit.

a. Place 2 padded splints along opposite sides of the entire injured arm and tie them to the upper and lower arm in 4 places without changing the angle of the elbow.
   OR

b. If no splints are available, wrap a pillow around the arm, centered at the elbow, and tie or pin it in place.

Breaks & Sprains
Forearm, wrist, hand & fingers

Important—read first:

Before immobilizing the injured area, keep movement to an absolute minimum.

Do not try to straighten the injured part.

If the skin over a suspected fracture is broken, do not touch it. Cover it with the cleanest available cloth.

Check for numb fingers periodically to be sure that a bandage is not too tight.

Seek medical attention immediately.

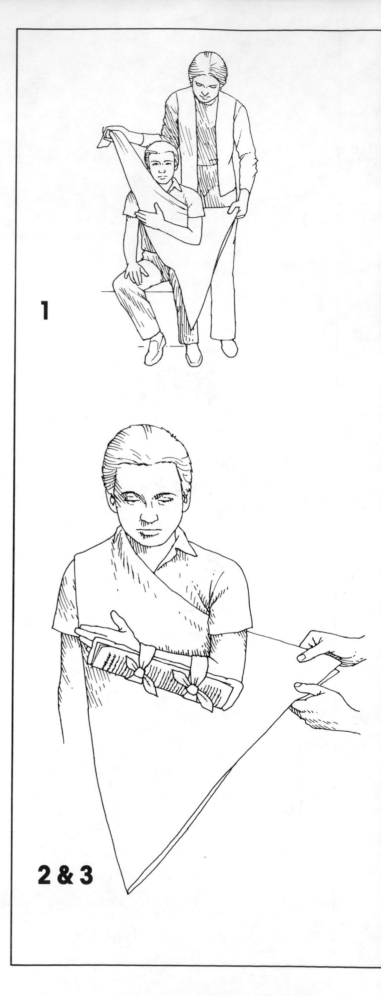

1

2 & 3

Doctor's comments:
   Forearm and wrist fractures are often the result of falls. The knuckles, especially on the little finger, are often broken in fistfights.
   Elevation of the injured part with a sling or by some other means is essential to prevent severe swelling.

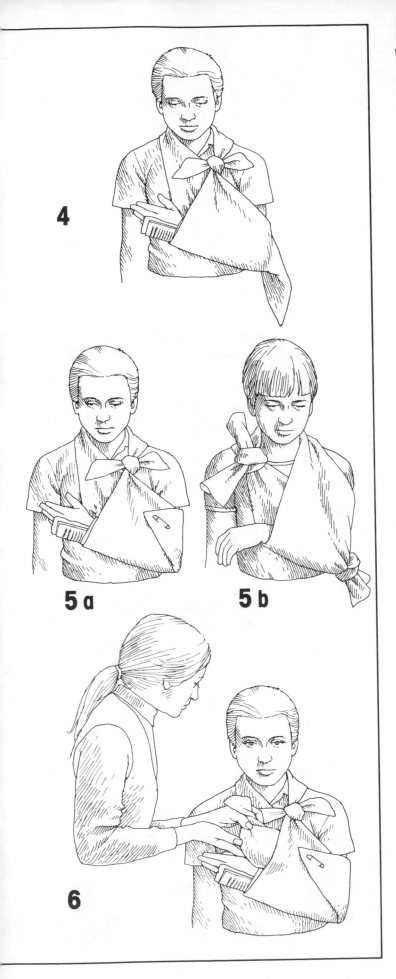

4

5 a

5 b

6

How to immobilize with a splint and sling

For any suspected injury to the bones or joints of the lower arm, wrist, hand, or fingers:

1. Place a large triangular bandage, or a shirt, on the person's chest, with one corner under the elbow of the injured arm, one corner over the other shoulder, and one corner down near the knees.

2. Place a padded splint around the injured arm extending from the elbow to the middle of the fingers so that they remain exposed. A large magazine, newspaper, or corrugated cardboard from a box makes a good three-sided splint, lined with cloth. Tie the splint in place at both ends of the forearm, but do not tie directly over the injury.

3. Place the arm gently across the person's chest at a right angle, with the hand about 4 inches above the elbow. The thumb should be pointing upward if this is comfortable.

4. Bring the lowest corner of the triangular bandage up over the shoulder on the injured side. Tie the two upper corners together. The knot should be on the side to avoid painful pressure on the neck.

5. Fold the third corner around the elbow of the injured arm and (a) pin it or (b) tie in place. Be sure the person's fingertips are not covered.

6. Gently apply ice wrapped in a cloth to decrease swelling. Check for numb fingers periodically; loosen bandages if necessary.

7. The person will probably be most comfortable sitting up while being transported to medical care.

Fingers:

It is not necessary to put a splint on an injured finger while awaiting medical care, even though it may be broken. If a finger joint is dislocated, attempting to splint it may cause harm.

Breaks & Sprains
Pelvis

Important—read first:

Call immediately for medical assistance to come to the scene. Internal bleeding is possible in cases of pelvic injury. Up to one-third of the blood volume can be lost when the pelvis is fractured.

Before immobilizing the injured area, keep movement to an absolute minimum.

If the skin over a suspected fracture is broken, do not touch it. Cover it with the cleanest available cloth.

Pain in the groin or lower abdomen when a person tries to move after an accident (often an automobile accident) may indicate a fracture of the pelvis. In such a case, move the person as little as possible and immobilize his legs.

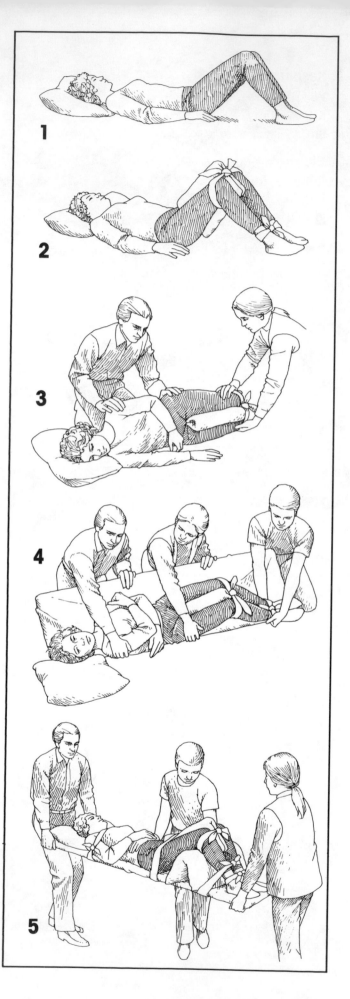

Doctor's comments:
Ideally, first aid is limited to immobilization of the legs, and trained personnel are called to the scene.

How to immobilize

1. Keep the person lying on his back. He will probably be more comfortable with both knees bent but may lie with both legs straight if he prefers.

2. Place a folded blanket or similar pad between the person's thighs, then tie his legs together at the knees and ankles to stabilize the injury. The knots should not press against his legs. Check ankle pulses periodically and check for numb toes to be sure that a bandage is not too tight.

3. Avoid transporting the person if at all possible. If professional help cannot come to you, roll the person onto his side using as many helpers as possible. Roll the pelvis and legs as a single unit.

4. Place a padded long board, door, or table leaf behind the person and roll him onto his back on top of it. Again, roll the pelvis and legs as a single unit.

5. Tie the person securely to the padded board and place a pillow in the space under his bent knees. Carry him gently on the board. Check pulse at both ankles periodically and check for numb toes; loosen ties if necessary.

Breaks & Sprains
Hip & upper leg

Important—read first:

Do not try to straighten the injured upper leg bone.

If the skin over a suspected fracture is broken, do not touch it. Cover it with the cleanest available cloth.

Before immobilizing the injured area, keep movement to an absolute minimum.

Call immediately for medical assistance to come to the scene.

With fractures of the femur, the injured leg often appears shortened, and the foot is usually turned outward. With dislocations of the hip joint, the thigh is often turned inward.

If professional assistance can be summoned, do not try to immobilize the leg or transport the person. Keep him lying down and make him as comfortable as possible.

If help cannot come to you and you must transport the person, immobilize the leg as instructed at right.

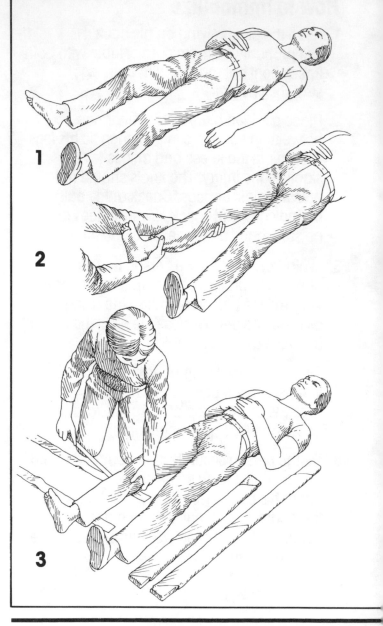

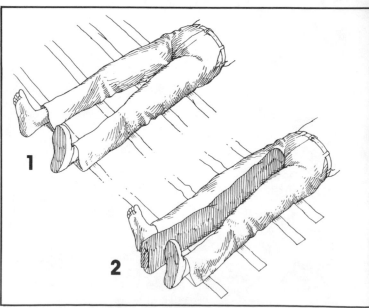

Doctor's comments:
Fractures of the femur are common in automobile accidents and in falls, particularly among the elderly. They cause severe pain in younger people but may only be slightly painful in the elderly.

Pain and resistance in the hip joint when you attempt to straighten the leg may indicate a dislocation of the hip, which is best treated in the same way as a fracture of the pelvis.

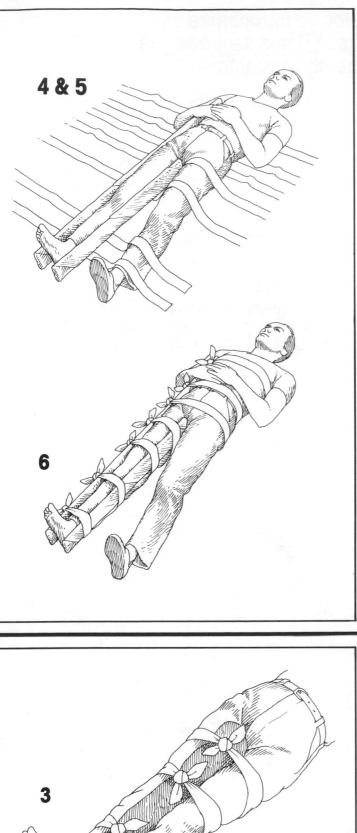

How to immobilize with splints

1. Keep the person lying down and make him as comfortable as possible.

2. If the injured leg is bent, slowly and gently try to straighten the knee. If you meet with resistance and pain in the hip joint, stop and treat as for a pelvis injury —see the preceding section, page 56.

3. If long boards, oars, straight branches, etc., are available, use them as splints. One splint should be long enough to reach from the crotch to past the heel. The other should reach from the armpit to past the heel. Wrap padding around both splints. Use a stick to push 7 long cloth strips under the hollows of the person's body: 1 under the ankle, 3 under the knee, and 3 under the lower back.

4. Slide the cloth strips into position: 1 under the ankle, 1 below the knee, 2 under the lower and upper thigh (but not at the level of the suspected break), 1 around the pelvis, 1 around the waist, and 1 below the armpits.

5. Place both splints next to the injured leg—the short splint on the inside, the long on the outside— on top of the cloth strips.

6. Tie the splints on snugly. The knots should not press against the leg. Check pulse at the ankle periodically and check for numb toes; loosen ties if necessary.

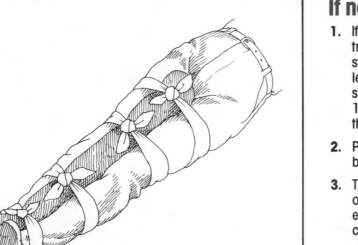

If no splints are available

1. If long splints are not available and the person must be transported, use a stick to push 4 long cloth strips under the hollows of the injured and uninjured legs: 1 under the ankles and 3 under the knees. Then slide the strips into position: 1 under the ankles, 1 below the knees, and 2 under the lower and upper thighs (but not at the level of the suspected break).

2. Place a folded blanket or similar thick padding between the person's legs.

3. Tie the person's legs together so that he can immobilize one with the other. Knots should not press against either leg. Check pulse at both ankles periodically and check for numb toes; loosen ties if necessary.

Breaks & Sprains
Knee

Important—read first:

Before immobilizing the injured knee, keep movement to an absolute minimum.

If the skin over a suspected fracture is broken, do not touch it. Cover it with the cleanest available cloth.

Check pulse at the ankle periodically and check for numb toes to be sure that a bandage is not too tight.

Seek medical attention immediately.

If an injured knee is bent, try very gently to straighten it.

If this is painful, leave the knee bent and follow the instructions at right (this page).

If the knee is straight or can be gently straightened, follow the instructions on the opposite page.

How to immobilize an injured knee if it is bent and you CANNOT gently straighten it

1. Leave it bent. With the person lying on his back or his uninjured side, have him bend his uninjured knee at the same angle as his injured knee. Place folded towels or other padding between his calves and between his thighs, with no padding against the knee. Tie his legs together at mid-calf and mid-thigh so that one leg can splint the other.

2. Gently apply ice wrapped in cloth to the knee to reduce the swelling. Check pulse at both ankles periodically and check for numb toes; loosen ties if necessary.

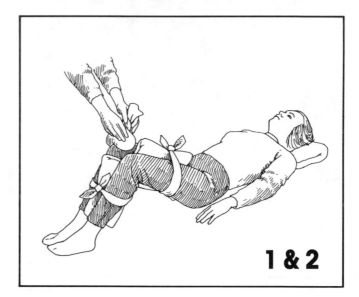

1 & 2

Doctor's comments:
Fractures of the kneecap and dislocations of the knee are both common athletic injuries and are difficult to tell apart. With a broken kneecap, the leg usually will be straight or can be straightened gently without severe pain or resistance. A long splint is then the best first-aid remedy. A dislocated knee cannot be straightened without pain and resistance, and it should be immobilized as is. Because a dislocated knee can cut off the blood supply to the lower leg, immediate medical care is absolutely essential.

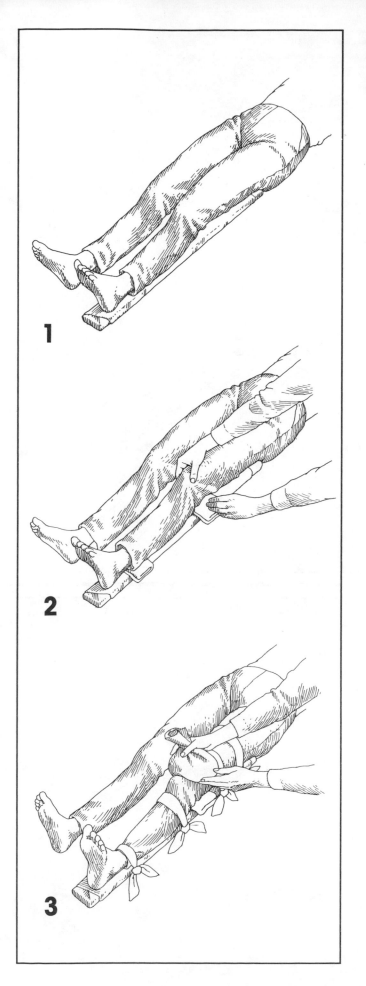

How to immobilize an injured knee if it is straight or if you CAN gently straighten it

1. Wrap padding around a board at least 4 inches wide. Ideally, the board should reach from the top of the thigh to past the heel. Gently place it under the injured leg.

2. Add padding to fill the hollows under the ankle and knee.

3. Tie the splint to the leg at the ankle, above and below the knee, and at the upper thigh. Do not tie over the knee itself. The knots should not press against the leg. Gently apply ice wrapped in cloth to the knee to reduce swelling. Check pulse at the ankle and check for numb toes; loosen ties if necessary.

Breaks & Sprains
Lower Leg

Important—read first:

Before immobilizing the injured area, keep movement to an absolute minimum.

Do not try to straighten the injured leg bones themselves.

If the skin over a suspected fracture is broken, do not touch it. Cover it with the cleanest available cloth.

Check pulse at the ankle periodically and check for numb toes to be sure that a bandage is not too tight.

Seek medical attention immediately.

If two boards, straight branches, or other materials for making splints are available, follow the instructions under "How to immobilize with splints" at top of opposite page.

If no splints are available, follow instructions at bottom of opposite page.

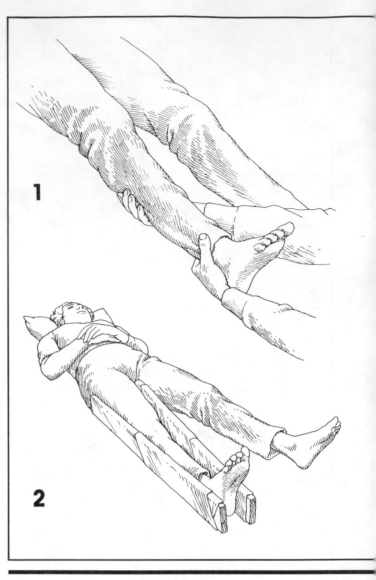

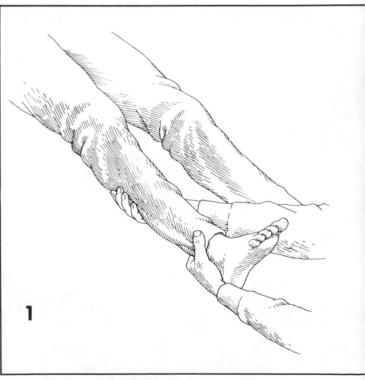

Doctor's comments:
    Pedestrians struck by automobile bumpers often suffer fractures of the lower leg. Since only a thin layer of skin covers the shin, open, or "compound," fractures are common; it is essential to keep them clean.

How to immobilize with splints

For all injuries of the lower leg bones, between the knee and the ankle:

1. Gently straighten the knee of the injured leg if it is bent.

2. If 2 boards, straight branches, or other objects suitable for splints are available, use them. Both boards must reach from well above the knee to past the heel. Wrap padding around both splints and place them along the inner and outer sides of the injured leg.

3. Tie the splints to the leg in 3 or 4 places. Do not tie directly over the injury. Knots should not press against the leg. Check pulse at the ankle periodically and check for numb toes; loosen ties if necessary.

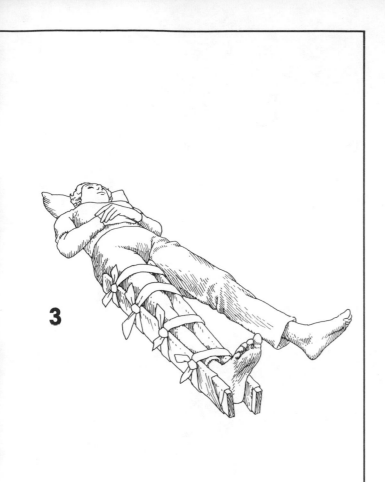

3

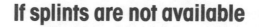

If splints are not available

1. Gently straighten the knee of the injured leg if it is bent.

2. Place a folded blanket or similar padding between the peron's legs, then tie his legs together in 3 or 4 places so that he can immobilize one leg with the other. Do not tie directly over the injury. Knots should not press against either leg.

3. Check pulses at both ankles periodically and check for numb toes; loosen ties if necessary.

4. The person will be most comfortable lying down while being transported to medical care.

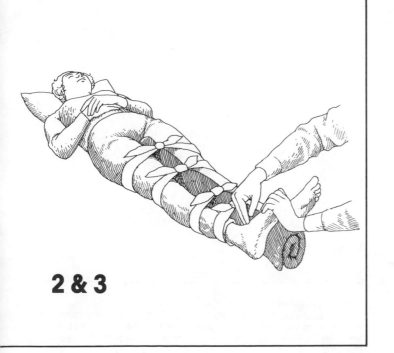

2 & 3

Breaks & Sprains
Ankle, foot & toes

Important—read first:

Before immobilizing the injured area, keep movement to an absolute minimum.

Do not try to straighten the injured part.

If the skin over a suspected fracture is broken, do not touch it. Cover it with the cleanest available cloth.

Check for numb toes periodically to be sure that a bandage is not too tight.

Seek medical attention immediately.

How to immobilize and reduce swelling

1. Do not let the person try to walk. Remove his shoe if possible, or at least loosen it.

2. Place a pillow under the lower calf with about one-third of it extending out past the heel. A folded blanket is almost as good.

3. Fold the upper two-thirds of the pillow around the ankle and tie it in place with 2 cloth strips.

4. Fold the lower third of the pillow around the foot and tie it in place with a cloth strip, leaving the toes exposed.

5. Elevate the foot to decrease swelling. Check periodically for numb toes; loosen ties if necessary. If a toe is injured, gently apply ice wrapped in cloth.

Toes:

Prompt application of ice will decrease swelling. Doctors rarely apply a splint or cast, even if the toe is broken. Pressure can be avoided by wearing an old shoe or sneaker with the end cut away. Consult a doctor to be sure additional foot injury has not occurred.

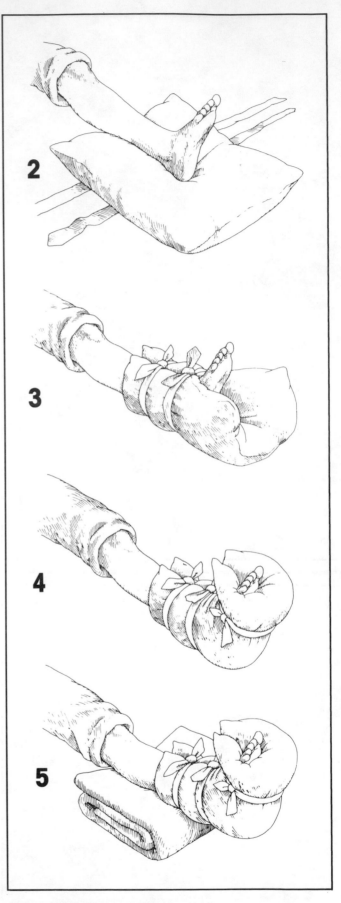

Doctor's comments:
Physicians usually need x-rays to tell a badly sprained ankle or foot from a fracture, so it is safest to treat such injuries as fractures. Even if the injury happens to be a sprain, it is not helpful to "walk on a sprain," as was previously believed.

Breathing
Problems

overview:

Cessation of breathing may result from a variety of mechanisms, including airway obstruction, lack of blood flow to the brain, drug overdose, etc.

The proper treatment involves training in CPR. It is beyond the scope of this book to instruct the reader in cardiopulmonary resuscitation. Once again, the authors urge you to enroll in a CPR course so that you will be prepared to use this lifesaving technique *properly* in the event of an emergency.

Breathing problems such as shortness of breath may be due to simple anxiety (hyperventilation) or serious heart disease. Reassurance can calm the person and end an episode of hyperventilation.

For shortness of breath related to heart or lung disease, other symptoms usually are present and indicate the need for immediate medical attention.

For **Choking,** see page 77.

66-67 **Shortness of breath** What to do for a person who is breathing rapidly and feels "out of breath"

68 **Croup (difficulty inhaling)** How to help a person who inhales loudly and with difficulty

Breathing Problems
Shortness of breath

Important—read first:

Shortness of breath may be due to heart or lung disease. Seek medical attention immediately if signs of possible heart failure or heart attack accompany shortness of breath:

- Pain in the chest, arm, shoulder, jaw, or upper abdomen
- Heavy perspiration, clammy skin even without exercise
- A history of heart problems or heart medications

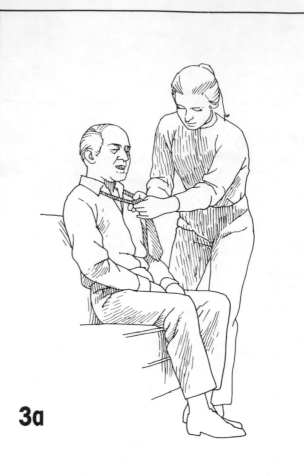

3a

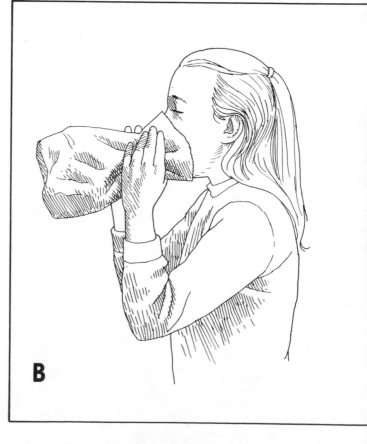

B

Doctor's comments:

Congestive heart failure is the most serious cause of shortness of breath. It occurs when the heart is not pumping efficiently, allowing fluid to back up into the lungs. This can be a chronic condition (with periodic flare-ups) in people with long-standing heart disease, or it can come on suddenly when the heart is weakened by a heart attack. In either case, emergency medical care is necessary.

Hyperventilation is often a frightening but harmless reaction to emotional upset or stress. Rapid breathing removes too much carbon dioxide from the body, causing symptoms such as dizziness and tingling, which in turn increase panic in a vicious cycle. Holding the breath or breathing the same air from a bag restores carbon dioxide, removes the symptoms, and makes it easier to calm the person. A hyperventilating person may faint. If this occurs, normal breathing will resume automatically.

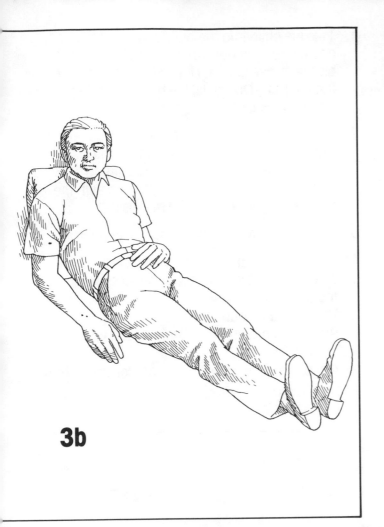

3b

For any shortness of breath

Do the following as soon as possible, whether or not danger signs of heart disease are present:

1. Look at the person to determine his age and whether he seems generally healthy.

2. Try to find out if the person has a history of heart or lung disease or takes any heart medications.

3. Have the person (a) sit up or (b) semi-recline (let him choose the more comfortable of the two positions). Loosen clothing around the neck, such as a tight collar or tie. Try to calm and reassure the person.

4. If: (a) the person's rate of breathing slows after you calm him; (b) there are no other symptoms such as pain in the chest, clammy skin, etc.; and (c) the circumstances indicate shortness of breath is due to anxiety, this probably is a case of hyperventilation. It is most common in young people.

5. If calming the person does not slow his rate of breathing, shortness of breath may be a symptom of an underlying heart or lung disease. Seek medical attention immediately.

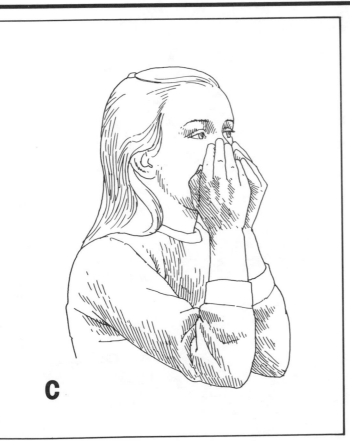

C

Controlling hyperventilation

A hyperventilating person usually responds to reassurance and to one of the following approaches:

A. Encourage the person to breathe slower and slower and to hold his breath for a few seconds before exhaling.

   OR

B. Have the person breathe the same air repeatedly for 3 or 4 minutes by breathing into a paper bag held over his mouth and nose, or into a bowl.

   OR

C. If there is no bag or other object to breathe into, have the person breathe into his own cupped hands.

Breathing Problems

Croup (difficulty inhaling)

Important—read first:

Do not put a spoon or other object in the mouth to look at the child's throat.

Seek medical attention immediately if any of these danger signs are present:

- ☐ Extreme difficulty breathing
- ☐ High fever or sudden rise in temperature
- ☐ Drooling

Sometimes infants or children with allergies or colds develop swelling in the throat that makes it difficult for them to inhale and causes a croaking sound when they breathe in. This condition is called croup and is often accompanied by hoarseness and a harsh cough.

The danger signs described above may be evidence of epiglottitis, which is a medical emergency. If there is any question or concern, contact your doctor.

1. Take the child into the bathroom, shut the door, and turn on the hot water in the shower full-blast to make steam. (If you have no shower, use the tub.) Do not let the hot water splash on the child, as it can scald him.

2. Sit the child up in a high place, such as on your shoulders, where he can breathe in the steam. Comfort the child and encourage him to breathe slowly. Stay in the bathroom with the hot water on for at least 20 minutes.

3. Put the child to bed with a vaporizer nearby.

4. Seek medical attention immediately if:
- ☐ Breathing gets worse, not better, despite the steam
- ☐ The croaking sound continues
- ☐ Prolonged breathing difficulties lead to exhaustion
- ☐ Any of the danger signs appear (see **Important** box at left)

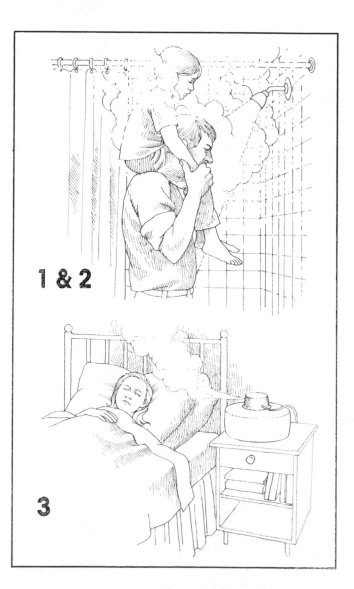

1 & 2

3

Doctor's comments:

Croup usually occurs in young children (it is rare in older children and adults). Most bouts of croup happen at night. With steam treatment and the use of a vaporizer, the symptoms usually subside to those of a mild cold. When croup does start during the day, it often gets worse at night; in this case, be prepared to seek medical assistance.

Burns

overview:

Treatment varies according to the severity, or "degree," of the burn. Try to identify the degree of the most severe part of the burn, usually in the center of the affected area, then see the appropriate section of this chapter. The symptoms of each degree are given at right to help you. **If you are unsure, treat for a third-degree burn.**

The treatment of burns caused by heat or electricity starts with cold water to cool tissue and keep tissue damage to a minimum—except with large third-degree burns (more than 2 inches across), where cold water can increase severity of shock.

As you treat burns, always remember that your goals are to relieve pain, prevent shock, and avoid contamination that could lead to infection.

Chemical burns present special problems. Flush immediately and thoroughly with water, then turn to **Chemical Burns,** page 74. For chemical burns of the eye, see **Eye Injuries,** page 107.

70-71 **First-degree burns:** red skin with mild swelling and pain

70-78 **Second-degree burns:** blisters on red, streaked, or blotchy skin, with swelling, a moist, oozing surface, and pain.

72-73 **Third-degree burns:** white or charred skin, often with little or no pain; all electrical burns

74 **Chemical burns**

Burns

First-degree burns: red skin with mild swelling and pain

Second-degree burns: blisters on red, streaked, or blotchy skin, with swelling, a moist, oozing surface, and pain.

Important—read first:

Rapid but proper first aid for burns is essential **before** medical care is at hand.

With burns of the face, or exposure to smoke in an enclosed space (inhalation of hot air or smoke) assume the presence of respiratory burns and seek medical attention immediately.

Do not open blisters or remove dead skin.

Do not remove clothing that sticks to burned area.

Do not put butter or household remedies on burns. Use pain-relief medicines, ointments, or sprays only on small first-degree burns or upon a doctor's instruction.

Do not press on a burned area.

Seek medical attention immediately for burns of the face, for extensive first-degree burns, and for all but minor second-degree burns.

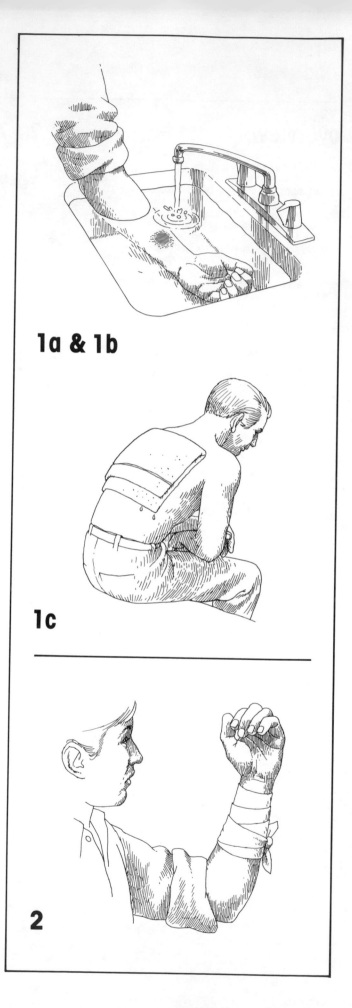

1a & 1b

1c

2

Doctor's comments:

First-degree burns involve only the outermost layer of the skin, which becomes red but not broken or blistered. Irritation of nerve endings in this layer produces pain that can be intense, but healing is usually rapid and complete. Common causes of first-degree burns are overexposure to the sun, and brief contact with hot objects. First degree burns can be treated at home by cooling the part with water, aspirin, oral fluids and aloe vera ointment.

Second-degree burns involve deeper layers of the skin, releasing body fluids that cause blisters. Pain is usually more severe, and shock is possible. Medical attention is necessary for relief of symptoms and care of blisters. Common causes of second-degree burns are deep sunburns, prolonged contact with hot objects, scalding with hot liquids and steam, and flash burns from flammable liquids such as gasoline. If a second degree burn covers a large area, see a doctor for advice on relieving pain and guarding against infection and dehydration. This is absolutely essential if more than 10 percent of the body (e.g., an entire leg or back) is burned.

Cold water, quickly applied, removes some excess heat from the skin and can prevent a burn from progressing to a more severe degree. It also provides considerable relief of pain, prevents swelling, and cleans the area, decreasing the chance of infection.

Butter and other household remedies are ineffective, may cause infection, and could require painful removal by a doctor in order for him to inspect and treat the burn.

First aid for first-degree and minor second-degree burns

Rapid but proper first aid for burns is essential. Minor second-degree burns are those small enough to be covered by a 2″ x 2″ dressing and not involving the face, hands, or feet.

1. Quickly cool the part with water.
a. Put the burned part under cold running water (not so forceful that it causes pain or breaks blisters).

    OR

b. Immerse the burned part in a sink full of cold water (do not use ice).

    OR

c. When a tap or sink is inconvenient, apply cold, wet compresses, using clean towels, handkerchiefs, or clothing.

2. Continue water treatment for 5 minutes or until pain subsides. Then gently pat dry with a sterile or clean cloth, and cover the burned area loosely with a sterile or clean dry cloth.

3. For second-degree burns of hands, feet, perineum, and face, and burns covering greater than 10 to 15 percent of the body (e.g., an entire leg or back), seek medical attention.

4. Also seek medical attention for burns which blister.

Burns

Third-degree burns: white or charred skin, often with little or no pain; all electrical burns

Important—read first:

Rapid but proper first aid for burns is essential **before** medical care is at hand.

With burns of the face, or exposure to smoke in an enclosed space (inhalation of hot air or smoke), assume the presence of respiratory burns and seek medical attention immediately.

With electrical burns:
> Look for both an entry and an exit burn—two burns on different parts of the body where electricity has gone in and come out—and treat both as third-degree burns.

Remove constricting clothing or jewelry.

Use cold water (not ice) on small third-degree burns.

Do not open blisters or remove dead skin.

Do not put butter or household remedies on burns or use pain-relief medication, ointments, or sprays without a doctor's instruction.

Do not press on the burned area.

Seek medical attention immediately for all third-degree burns.

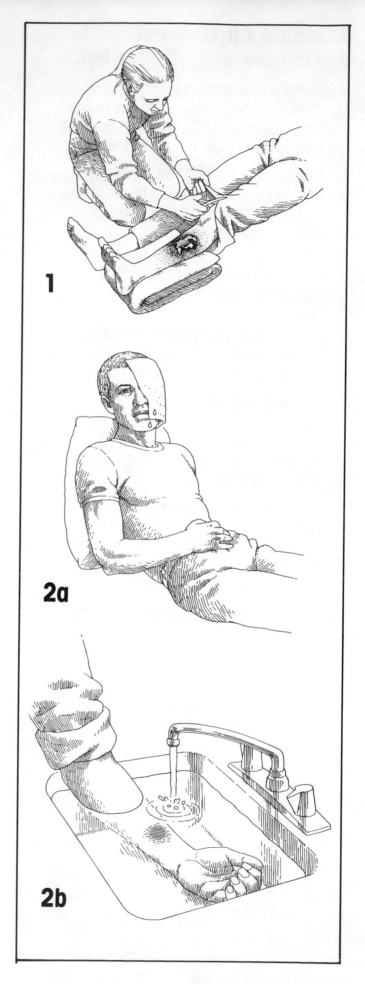

1

2a

2b

Doctor's comments:

Third-degree burns involve actual destruction of all layers of the skin and may require grafting in order for it to heal. Because the nerve endings have been destroyed, there may be little or no pain. Never let a person walk on a burned foot, even if he insists that it is not painful.

Third-degree burns are usually caused by fire or electric shock. A small third-degree burn may be hard to see in the middle of a larger area of second- and first-degree skin damage. For this reason, when in doubt, treat for a third-degree burn.

Shock is a major problem in third-degree burns. Cold water should not be used if the burn is large, more than 2 inches across, since too-sudden cooling can increase the severity of shock. Medical care is essential, even for the smallest third-degree burns.

First aid for third-degree burns

1. Remove constricting clothing or jewelry, which may become tighter if swelling occurs.

2. Quickly cool the part with water.

a. Apply cold, wet compresses with a clean cloth.
Observe closely for breathing problems.

OR

b. With small third-degree burns (less than 2 inches across), put the burned part under cold running water or in a sink of cold water, or apply cold wet compresses, for 5 minutes. Do not use ice. Pat dry and cover with a sterile or clean dry cloth.

3. Cover with a dressing.

4. Proper dressing of third-degree burns of the fingers or toes requires separating the burned fingers or toes so they do not adhere to each other. This is best done by trained medical personnel.

5. Seek medical assistance immediately and treat for shock if you are properly trained.

Burns
Chemical burns

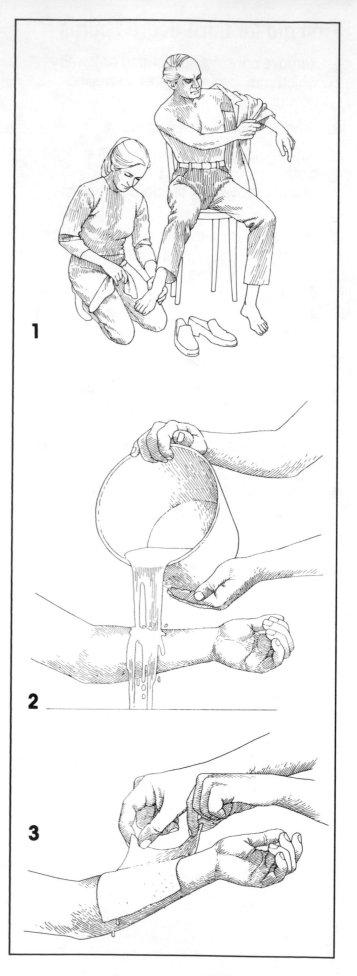

1. Remove contaminated clothing, including shoes and socks.

2. Flush the burned area immediately with large quantities of cool water from a shower, hose (not too forceful), faucet, or pail. Continue flushing for at least 5 full minutes.

3. Relieve pain with cool, wet compresses while awaiting medical care.

4. Cover the burn with a moist dressing.

5. Even if the burned area is not large, seek medical attention.

Doctor's comments:
The substance causing a chemical burn must be removed as quickly as possible. Water dilutes it and flushes it away, and removal of clothing takes any absorbed chemicals away from the skin.

Attempts to neutralize an acid with an alkali or vice versa are unwise. The two react chemically, causing heat and additional burning.

Frequently encountered household products that cause third-degree chemical burns include rust removers (hydrofluoric acid), commercial grade acids (nitric, sulfuric, phosphoric), and cement and drain cleaners (hydrochloric acid in sufficient strength). These must be used with caution.

Chest Injuries

overview:

Significant injuries to the chest carry the possibility of broken ribs, chest instability, lung injury, fluid or air in the lung cavity. Shortness of breath and pain on breathing may result. This is a life-threatening situation. Therefore, persons with chest injuries need immediate medical attention. Definitive treatment is available only in a hospital.

If you encounter a person with significant injuries who has shortness of breath and pain on breathing, this may indicate serious injury of the chest wall, lungs, heart, or of the blood vessels of the chest. Seek immediate medical attention.

An open chest wound in a small child can be fatal. Cover it with your hand to seal it until help arrives.

Do not remove impaled objects.

By definition, chest injuries are serious and beyond the bounds of first aid by a lay person.

Your immediate priority is to find expert medical help.

Choking &
Swallowed Objects

overview:

If a person seems to be choking, the first step is to decide if first aid is necessary. If he can breathe, cough forcefully, or speak (or if a baby can cry), do not give first aid but watch closely and be prepared to help.

If the person cannot do any of these (which means he has a completely blocked airway), or if he can only cough faintly and breathe noisily with great difficulty, do give first aid. Proper treatment combines blows to the back and pressure to the abdomen (the Heimlich Maneuver). Turn to the appropriate section—for a conscious adult or an infant—and follow the instructions carefully. Acute airway obstruction from aspirating food or foreign objects is life-threatening. First aid requires CPR training. You are urged to enroll in a CPR course and learn how to deal with airway obstructions.

If an object has been swallowed (not lodged in the breathing passages), there is no appropriate first aid. Seek medical assistance immediately.

78-79 Conscious adult or child (over age 1)

80-81 Infant (up to age 1)

82 Swallowed objects

Choking
Conscious adult or child (over age 1)

Important—read first:

Recognize choking by

- ☐ inability to talk
- ☐ noisy, difficult breathing (crowing respiration)
- ☐ universal choking signal

Take a CPR course to learn how to help a choking victim. In the meantime, back blows and the Heimlich maneuver will be useful in some situations.

Do not try to pull any object from a choking person's mouth by forcing the mouth open and looking inside.

Suspect choking when a person who is eating or a child who is playing with small objects

- ☐ Suddenly collapses
- ☐ Grasps his throat
- ☐ Wheezes or coughs

If a person appears to be choking but can breathe and cough forcefully, be ready to assist if the situation gets worse— but do not give first aid yet. The person's own coughing is more effective than anything a first-aider can do.

If the person is not coughing strongly, ask, "Can you speak?" If he can speak, do not give first aid.

If he cannot speak, give first aid as described on the opposite page.

Doctor's comments:

First aid for choking, including abdominal thrusts (the "Heimlich Maneuver"), is one of the most important advances in emergency care in the past decade.

Choking occurs most often while eating. It frequently involves older adults who are eating meat and chewing it poorly. They may be drinking alcohol, wearing uncomfortable dentures, or just talking with their mouths full. In the past, sudden collapse in this situation was often mistaken for a heart attack (a "café coronary"), and lives were lost that could have been saved.

Two methods are used to remove an object from the throat. Sometimes back blows work, sometimes thrusts work. The two together have a high success rate.

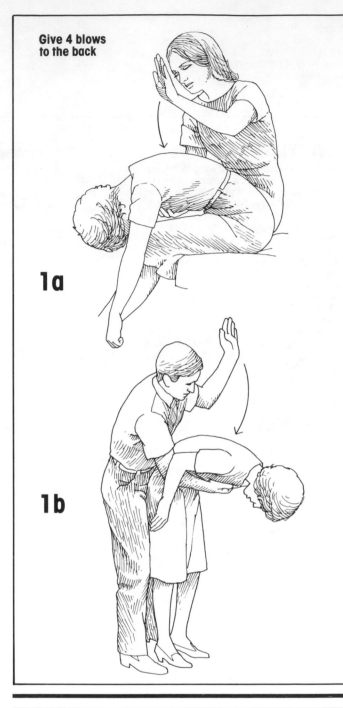

Give 4 blows to the back

1a

1b

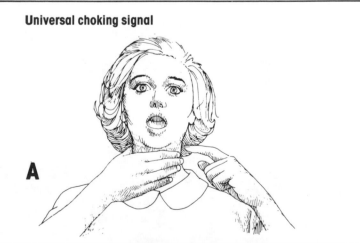

Universal choking signal

A

First aid for choking

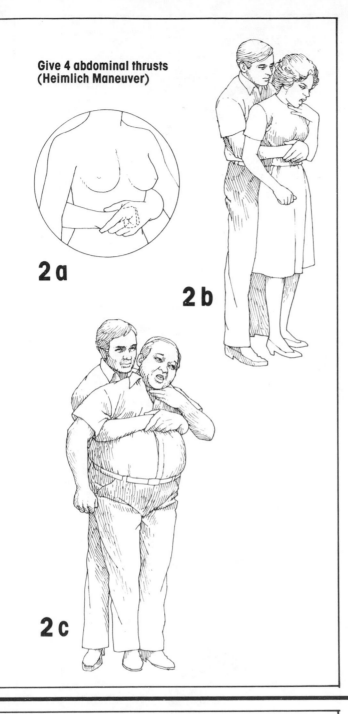

**Give 4 abdominal thrusts
(Heimlich Maneuver)**

2 a

2 b

2 c

1. Stand behind the person, who may be (a) seated or (b) standing. Support his chest with one hand and bend him forward so that his head is lower than his chest. Give 4 blows to his back, between the shoulder blades. Use the heel of your hand, and hit rapidly and hard enough to knock the object loose.

2. If the person continues to choke, put both arms around him and perform the "Heimlich Maneuver":

a. Press the thumb-side of one fist against his abdomen, halfway between his waist and the bottom of his ribs.

b. Grasp your fist with your other hand and give 4 quick, hard, inward and upward thrusts. Adjust the force of your thrusts to the person's size, especially important if you are treating a child.
OR

c. If extreme obesity or advanced pregnancy makes this impossible, give thrusts inward against the middle of the person's breastbone.

DON'T GIVE UP—CONTINUE THE CYCLE
If thrusts don't work, repeat 4 blows to the back, then 4 thrusts again. Have someone call for medical assistance while you continue the cycle until

☐ The object is dislodged and normal breathing begins. Stop first aid.
OR

☐ The person begins to cough forcefully. Stop first aid.
OR

☐ The person loses consciousness. This situation requires training in CPR.

If YOU are choking, give a signal

A. Let other people know. Give them an unmistakable signal by clutching your throat with one hand. This is the universally recognized sign of choking.

If you are alone and choking

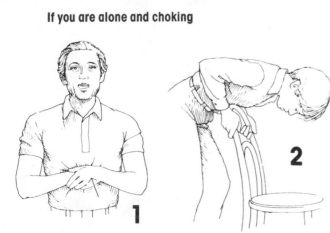

If you are alone and choking

1

2

1. You can perform the Heimlich Maneuver on yourself.
OR

2. You can push against your abdomen by leaning over the back of a chair or other blunt object.

Choking
Infant (up to age 1)

Important—read first:

Do not try to pull any object from a choking infant's mouth by forcing the mouth open and looking inside.

If a baby appears to be choking but can breathe, cry, or cough forcefully, be ready to assist if the situation gets worse, but do not give first aid yet. The baby's own coughing is more effective than anything a first-aider can do.

If the baby is not coughing strongly, give first aid as described on the opposite page.

Doctor's comments:
   Choking is a common childhood emergency that occurs when infants and young children put small toys or other objects in their mouths. Counteract this natural but dangerous form of curiosity by keeping small objects out of the reach of children. Also avoid larger playthings with small, removable parts.

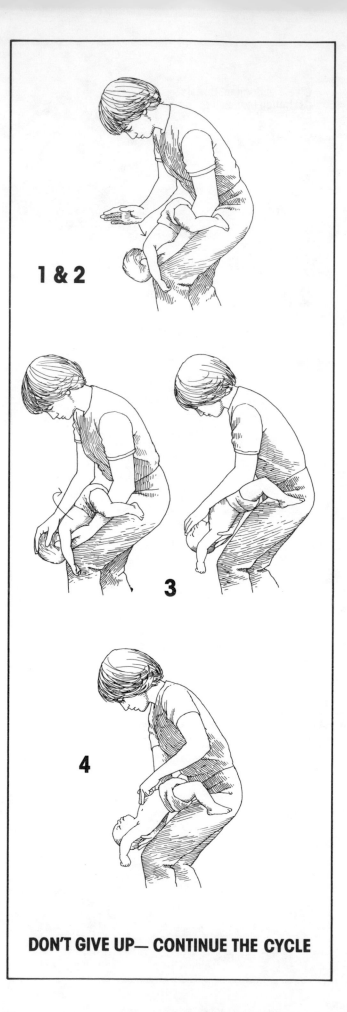

1 & 2

3

4

DON'T GIVE UP— CONTINUE THE CYCLE

When a baby is choking and conscious

1. Lay the baby face-down on your forearm, with your hand supporting his head. The baby's head should be lower than his chest.

2. Give 4 quick blows to his back between the shoulder blades. Use the heel of your hand.

3. Turn the baby over. Place your free hand on the back of the baby's head and hold him between your two forearms. Turn him face-up, with his head still lower than his body.

4. Put 2 fingertips on the baby's chest between the nipples. Press quickly and fairly hard 4 times.

5. If the baby continues to choke, repeat 4 blows, 4 presses. **DON'T GIVE UP.** If breathing stops and you are properly trained, use CPR.

Choking
Swallowed objects

If a child swallows a smooth object,
such as a coin or a marble, or an adult
swallows a larger smooth object,
there may be temporary discomfort as the
object passes through the esophagus
(the narrowest part of the digestive tract),
but usually there will be no difficulty
breathing. This is not true choking. If the
discomfort goes away, nothing need
be done. The object will pass through the
rest of the digestive tract harmlessly,
except for possible momentary discomfort
as it passes through the anus. No
x-rays or other medical procedures are
necessary, although your physician
should at least be notified about the event.

If, however, the pain persists for more than
5 minutes, the person is drooling, or
if a sharp object (fish bone, chicken bone)
seems to be lodged in the esophagus,
or if a dangerous object, such as a pin, has
been swallowed, seek medical
assistance. Pointed, nondigestible objects
like pins may need to be located
with x-rays and removed by a physician.

Common Injuries
(Soft Tissue Injuries)
Cuts, Bruises, & Minor Injuries

overview:

Common soft tissue injuries which can be treated by first aid alone and do not require medical attention include: scraping (abrasion), tearing (laceration), cutting (incision), and bruising. As long as they involve only the skin, are less than 1/2 inch long, do not gape or bleed freely, and are not associated with numbness or inability to move, pain, or penetration, these injuries can be cared for using simple first aid measures. In most cases, this means washing and scrubbing (irrigating) the injury with mild soap and water and then covering it with a clean (preferably sterile) dressing.

The first priority in face and jaw injuries is keeping breathing passages clear, followed by gentle control of bleeding and immobilization of possible lower-jaw fractures.

Soft tissue injuries which may need medical attention include injuries to the hands, fingers, feet, and toes. Such injuries carry a greater disability because of the special functions and anatomy of the tissues involved. Any hand injury associated with loss of motion or sensation or involving the nail or nailbed should receive medical attention.

For any soft tissue injury larger than 1 cm, which gapes, bleeds freely, and is associated with loss of motion or sensation, or with pain on motion, proper medical attention will speed healing.

84-85 **Minor cuts, scrapes & splinters**

86 **Bandaging minor cuts & scrapes—types of bandages**

87 **Bruises**

88-89 **Impaled objects**

90-91 **Face & jaw**

92 **Fishhook in the skin**

Common Injuries
(Soft tissue injuries)
minor cuts, scrapes & splinters

Important—read first:

Before you attend to minor cuts and scrapes, look for additional, not readily apparent injuries that may have occurred.

A tetanus booster is advisable with any wound, no matter how small, if none has been received within 10 years.

Prevent infection by washing minor cuts and scrapes.

Washing and scrubbing the cut or scrape clean with soap and water is especially important when there is tattooing of a scrape (e.g., gravel in the wound). Vigorous washing with soap and a sterile gauze pad usually remove superficial or slightly embedded material. If embedded material persists despite this, in a cosmetically important area (e.g., the face), seek medical attention. In other areas of the body, scrub the dirt out immediately (a soft toothbrush works well) using mild soap. Otherwise, the skin will be tattooed and infection is more likely.

Cover all scrapes and cuts with a clean, preferably sterile, dressing (e.g., Band-Aid,® gauze, telfa). This will relieve pain as well as prevent infection. Leave the dressing on, changing it once a day or sooner if it gets wet or dirty. Leaving a cut or scrape open to the air makes it more painful and delays healing. Ointments and creams are usually unnecessary and can be damaging if used. Follow instructions at right.

Doctor's comments:
With all soft tissue injuries it is important to know whether tetanus immunization is up to date (whether the person received tetanus toxoid within the past 10 years). If the person is in military service or received his school immunizations, it is likely that he has had a tetanus shot.

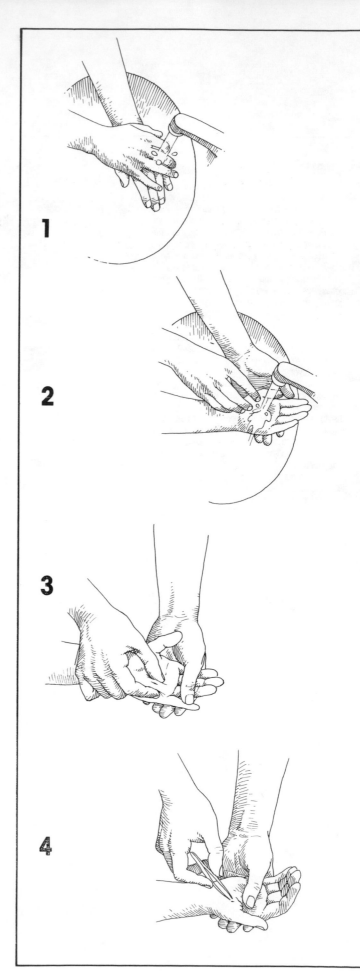

1

2

3

4

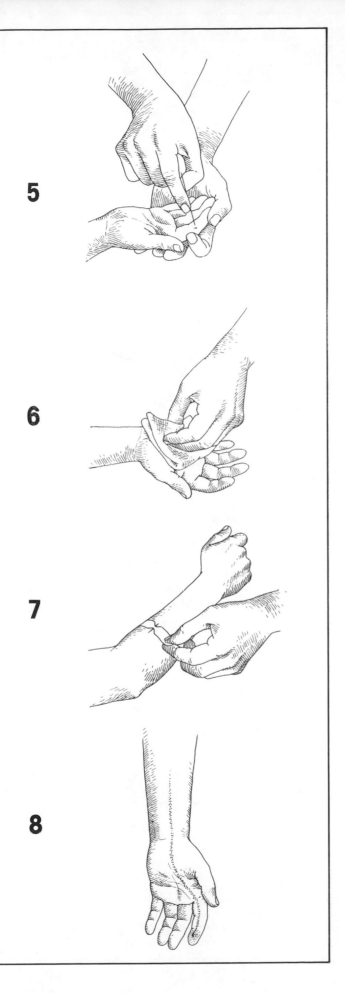

Prevent infection

1. First, scrub your hands with soap and water.

2. Next, wash the cut or scrape with soap and water to remove dirt. Be vigorous if necessary.

3. To clean a minor puncture wound, it may be necessary to encourage a little bleeding with gentle pressure.

4. Small particles and splinters near the surface of the skin may be removed with tweezers that have been sterilized (boiled or held over a flame, then allowed to cool). Do not remove large or deeply embedded objects.

5. Difficult-to-remove particles and splinters often can be teased out with a sterilized pin or needle. Pull them out at the same angle at which they went in.

6. Flush the scrape or cut with clean running water or poured water. Pat the wound dry, as rubbing may re-start the bleeding.

7. If the edges of a cut gape open, pull them together with a butterfly strip or a narrow piece of adhesive tape. For bandaging tips, see the next page.

8. Look for signs of infection, which may appear within hours or days. These include tenderness, throbbing, pus, redness, swelling around the wound, red streaks leading from it, swollen glands, and fever. If one or more of these signs appears, seek medical attention.

Common Injuries
(Soft tissue injuries)
Bandaging minor cuts & scrapes—types of bandages

Important—read first:

Whenever you have wrapped a bandage around an arm or leg, check periodically for a pulse farther out on the limb. If you feel no pulse, loosen the bandage a bit.

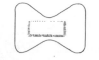

1. Fingertip strip:
Goes over the end of a finger or toe.

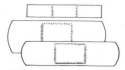

2. Adhesive strips:
Choose one large enough to cover the entire cut without unnecessarily limiting the movement of nearby joints.

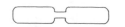

3. Butterfly strip:
Used to pull the edges of a cut together for healing.

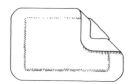

4. Four-sided bandage:
For larger cuts and scrapes.

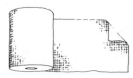

5. Knuckle bandage:
Covers the knuckle, but allows the finger to bend freely.

6. Non-stick gauze pad:
For use on even larger scrapes and wounds. (Several can be used together to apply direct pressure on a wound or to stabilize an impaled object.)

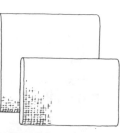

7. Adhesive tape:
(preferably hypo-allergenic): Used to secure gauze pads to flat surfaces. Can be substituted for a butterfly strip.

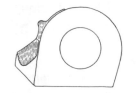

8. Gauze roll:
Used to secure gauze pads in place. (They are too narrow to be used as tourniquets.)

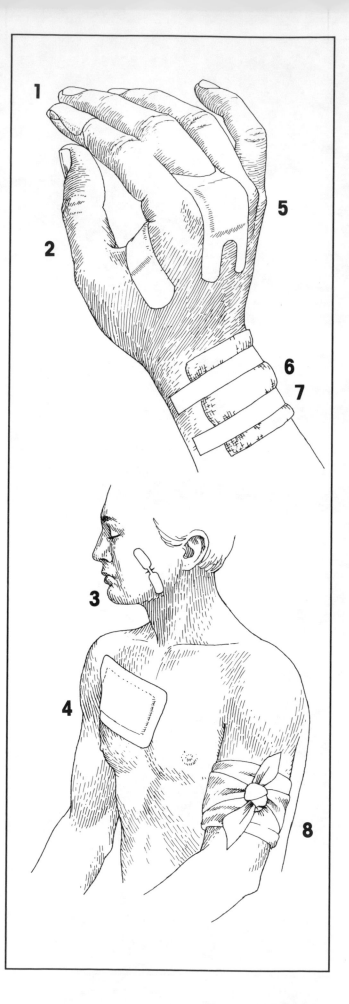

Doctor's comments:
Minor scrapes and scratches heal up to twice as fast when covered. Especially if they are in areas that are likely to be reinjured or to get dirty, they should be covered. All larger scrapes and cuts also should be covered.

When it is time for adhesive strips and tape to come off, you can make removal a little less painful by first applying some baby oil or mineral oil to the bandage and allowing it to soak in.

Common Injuries
(Soft tissue injuries)
Bruises

Important—read first:

Seek medical attention if pain and swelling become worse (indicating a possible bone or joint injury), or if the person seems to bruise easily and repeatedly.

Bruises are the most common of all injuries. Prompt first aid and follow-up care can make them less painful.

1. Quickly apply ice wrapped in cloth to the bruise.

2. Elevate the bruised part above the level of the person's heart. Keep it elevated 10–15 minutes for a small, mild bruise and an hour or two if the bruise is extensive and severe.

3. If the bruise remains tender or unsightly 24 hours after the injury, speed healing by applying warm, wet compresses.

   Bruises associated with joint injury—discoloration and swelling of the joint which limits motion—require medical attention. With all other bruises, first aid treatment using ice limits bleeding into the bruise and the swelling this causes—if applied within the first half hour.

Common Injuries
(Soft tissue injuries)
Impaled objects

Important—read first:

For impaled fishhooks, see page 92.

Do not remove an impaled object—anything may penetrate deeper than the skin, or into the abdomen or chest. Instead, stabilize the object to prevent further damage.

Do not move the injured person off a stationary impaling object.

Call for medical assistance immediately.

Control bleeding by applying direct pressure to the wound.

Stabilize the impaled object as described on the following page.

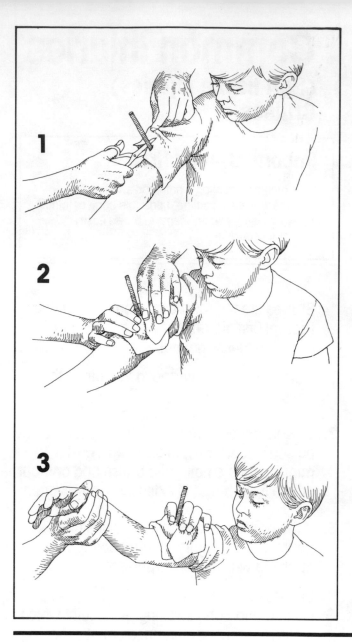

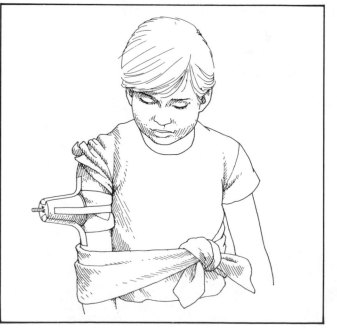

Doctor's comments:

Impaled objects include nails, arrows, large slivers of glass or wood, and any other objects that extend—or may extend—below the skin. Any movement of such objects can cause additional damage or bleeding. For this reason, removal of the object is dangerous and its stabilization extremely important.

Always seek medical attention immediately for removal of an impaled object, as well as for additional care and a tetanus booster, if one has not been received within the last 10 years. Tetanus infection can result from any wound, but it is more frequent in wounds caused by impaled objects because the tetanus bacteria grow best where there is little or no air.

Puncture wounds which penetrate beneath the skin have a high likelihood of getting infected. Seek medical attention especially if redness, tenderness, or pain develops at the site of injury. All puncture wounds of the feet, puncture wounds that go through clothing (leaving cloth fibers in the wound) or that leave other materials (such as wood slivers, glass, or thorns) in the wound, and those that result from dirty instruments should be seen by a physician. The risk of infection is very high in these cases. In addition, any puncture wound which becomes red and painful, that was not treated by a physician initially, requires medical attention.

Direct pressure

1. Carefully cut away clothing from around the impaled object.

2. Apply a bulky gauze or cloth dressing around the impaled object, covering the entire wound. Press firmly around the object and on the entire wound.

3. As you press around the impaled object, raise the wound above the level of the person's heart, if possible, but do not elevate a fractured limb.

How to stabilize an impaled object

1. Cover the wound with a dressing.

2. Poke a hole in the bottom of a paper cup and gently push it over the impaled object.

3. Use cloths, cardboard, or newspaper bolsters if no paper cup is available.

4. Tape the cup, cloths or newspaper securely in place. This stabilizes the impaled object.

5. If the impaled object is in an arm, fix that extremity to the body to stabilize the object. If the impaled object is in a leg, fix that leg to the uninvolved leg and to a backboard (wooden pole, etc.), if possible. This will stabilize the object.

Common Injuries
(Soft tissue injuries)
Face & jaw

Important—read first:

Check for neck injuries after any severe blow to the face. If the person is conscious, ask if he is aware of pain in the neck, paralysis, weakness, numbness or tingling of an arm or leg; if he is unconscious and a pinprick to each palm does not cause a reflex movement, suspect a neck injury. Go directly to Step A (on the opposite page) and treat as indicated.

Do not remove impaled objects.

Seek medical assistance immediately.

First aid for a face or jaw injury depends on the seriousness of the injury, whether the person is conscious or unconscious, and whether there are signs of a neck injury.

Face or jaw injury often is associated with a higher incidence of neck injury. If the person cannot breathe or is choking, turn him on his side. Try to keep his neck immobile by "log rolling" him (see page 18).

When the injury is **not serious**

If the person has a minor cut or scrape on the face, is conscious, and has no signs of neck injury, turn to **Bleeding,** page 23, and treat as described.

When the injury is **serious**

Call for medical assistance at once and keep the person warm.

Keep breathing passages open by placing the person in one of the positions described in Step A or B at right—lying down or sitting, whichever applies.

Gently control bleeding with direct pressure (C).

Treat for a possible broken jaw if necessary (D).

If medical help can't come to you, transport the person to an emergency room (E).

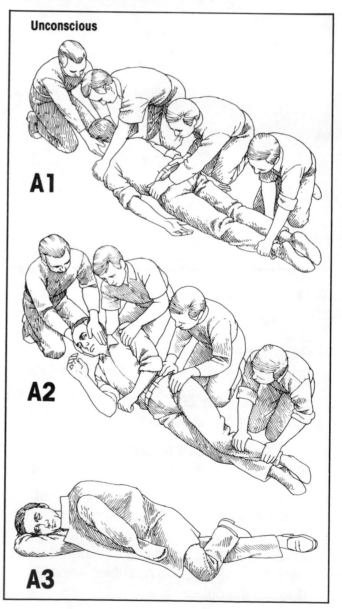

Unconscious

A1

A2

A3

Doctor's comments:

Your primary concern in serious face injuries is obstruction of the air passages by swelling, teeth or dentures, blood, saliva, vomit, or foreign matter. Removing these items from the mouth and positioning the person for drainage are the most important procedures.

When controlling bleeding, which is rarely severe in face injuries, you must apply pressure gently because fragile facial bones beneath the cut may be broken.

If an oral surgeon must wire a broken jaw or repair broken bones around the mouth, the person's dentures give him clues to the proper alignment. Teeth that have been knocked loose can often be reimplanted if they are kept moist. This is why it is important to take dentures and loose teeth with you to the emergency room.

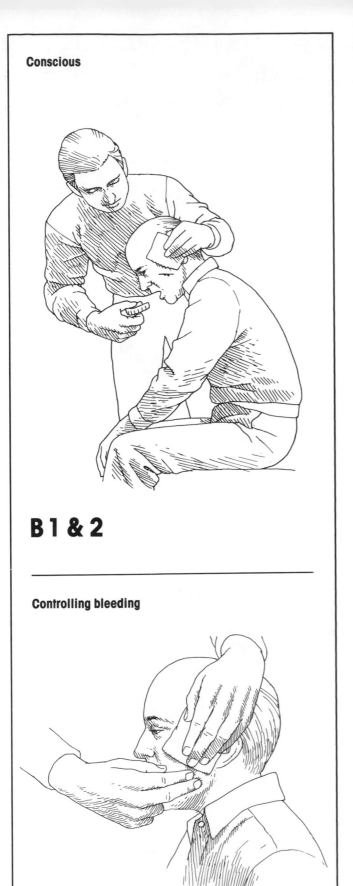

Conscious

B 1 & 2

Controlling bleeding

C 1

First aid for any serious face or jaw injury

A. If the person is unconscious OR is choking or cannot breathe and has signs of a neck injury:

1. Roll the person onto his side to clear breathing passages. Use at least 2 people—more, if possible—one holding his head, another holding his shoulders.

2. When the person holding the head says "go," roll all parts together, slowly and gently, keeping the head, neck, and torso unchanged in relation to each other.

3. When the person is on his side, provide support to keep his head and neck in the same unchanged positions.

4. Remove broken teeth, dentures, and any foreign matter from the mouth. Save dentures and any whole teeth.

B. If the person is conscious and has no signs of neck injury:

1. Remove broken teeth, dentures, and any foreign matter from the mouth. Save dentures and any whole teeth.

2. Sit the person up leaning forward so that blood and saliva can drain from his mouth.

C. After positioning the person (as in Step A or B), control bleeding:

1. Cover the wound completely with a sterile or clean cloth pad, and press gently on the entire pad.

2. If gentle pressure over the wound does not control bleeding, press more firmly.

D. For a possible broken jaw:

Signs of a fracture of the lower jaw include tenderness, swelling, a change in shape, pain upon moving the jaw, and loss of function (speaking, opening and closing the mouth). If a jaw fracture is suspected, seek medical attention.

E. Transportation:

If there are any signs of a neck injury, keep the person's head and neck immobile, and do not move him. (If medical help is hours away, take emergency transportation procedures described in **Back & Neck Injuries**, page 19.)

If there is no neck injury and help cannot come to you, transport the person to an emergency room—still lying on his side if unconscious, sitting up if conscious.

Take any dentures, whole or broken, with you to the hospital. Wrap any whole teeth that have come loose in wet sterile or clean cloth and take them with you as well.

Common Injuries
(Soft tissue injuries)
Fishhook in the skin

Important—read first:

Do not try to remove a fishhook from the face or from an eye.

Do not try to remove an embedded hook by pulling it back the way it went in.

Removing a fishhook

1. If only the point of the fishhook—not the barb—is in the skin, you can safely back it out.

2. If the barb is embedded, removal by a professional is advisable.

3. If prompt medical assistance is not available, push the hook farther in, in a shallow curve, until the point comes out through the skin.

4. Cut off the barbed end with a clipper or pliers.

5. Then back the shank of the hook out through the entry wound.

Preventing infection

6. After removing the hook, wash the area with soap and water, and cover it with a BAND-AID® Brand Adhesive Bandage or gauze bandage.

7. Consult a physician for further care.

Doctor's comments:
With any puncture wound, a tetanus booster is important if none has been received within the last 10 years.

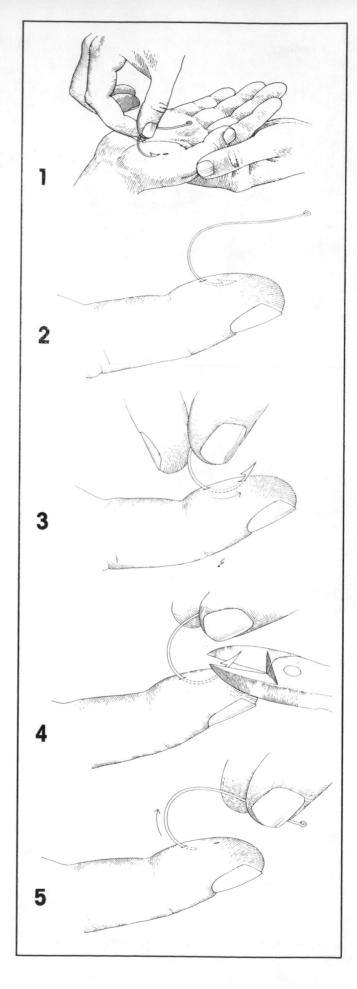

Convulsions
(Seizures, fits)

overview:

Seizures are not nearly as serious as they appear to be. While there is no first-aid measure that will stop them, complications can be minimized. Injury, often incurred when a convulsing person falls or thrashes about, can be prevented by catching him if he falls and removing hard or sharp objects from the immediate area. Choking while unconscious can be avoided by properly positioning the person.

For convulsions in young children with a high fever, give a sponge bath and aspirin or acetaminophen, in addition to the above measures, and seek medical assistance.

Turn immediately to p. 94.

Convulsions
(Seizures, fits)

Important—read first:

Do not restrain a convulsing person.

Do not try to put anything in a convulsing person's mouth, including your fingers.

Do not give the person anything to eat or drink until the episode is entirely over.

Do not throw water in the person's face.

In a "grand mal" or major seizure the person first loses consciousness then falls to the ground and has grunting or snorting respiration. He may foam at the mouth. Forceful jerking motions of the arms and legs (on one or both sides) appear and the person may lose bladder or bowel control. This type of seizure usually lasts 30 to 90 seconds.

Other kinds of seizures include "absence" seizures or "petit mal" where the person fades out for 30 to 60 seconds, or "focal seizures" where one part of the body moves in a jerking or twitching motion and the person seems unaware.

It is not necessary to call for medical assistance when a person has a seizure *unless* the seizure lasts longer than 2 minutes or there is repetitive seizure activity (more than one seizure per hour), indicating the possibility of major medical problems.

No first-aid measure can stop a seizure, but you can minimize the two major causes of complications by making sure the person does not injure himself and does not choke on anything in his mouth.

In children under age 6, the most common cause of seizures is sudden high fever. These so-called febrile convulsions are not usually a sign of serious illness. Treat as for any convulsion, and give a sponge bath and aspirin or acetaminophen to help prevent recurrence.

Doctor's comments:

Convulsions in themselves rarely do harm, but they may represent serious underlying disease requiring medical attention. In adults and children over age 6, convulsions are usually due to epilepsy. The cause of epilepsy in a given person is often unknown, but proper medical care can usually prevent repeated seizures or make them much less frequent. Seizures can also follow head injury, poisoning, electric shock, heat stroke, certain infectious diseases, hyperventilation, poisonous bites and stings, and drug use. They can also be caused by brain tumors or strokes.

The most important first-aid principles for convulsions are the "do not's." Restraining a person during a seizure may cause a fracture or torn muscle. Trying to separate his teeth and hold down his tongue is not necessary and could result in broken teeth or a broken finger—yours. Some people believe that giving a convulsing person a drink or throwing cold water in his face will "bring him out of it." It won't, but it could make him choke.

After a seizure has ended, disperse any crowd and shield the awaking person from onlookers to prevent embarrassment.

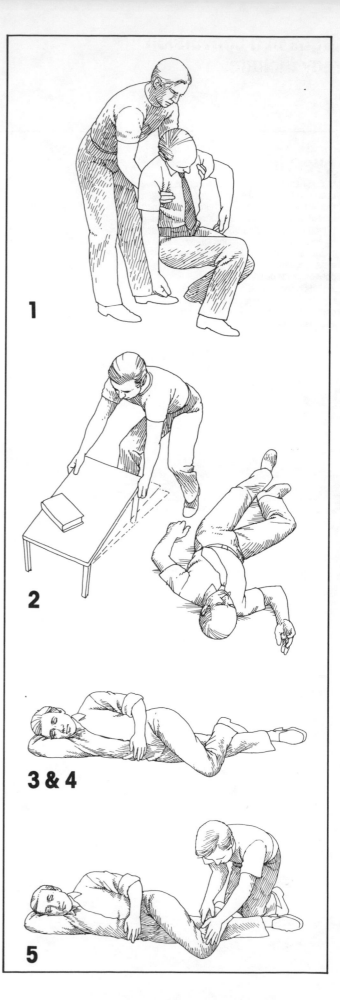

1

2

3 & 4

5

Signs of a convulsion may include:

- ☐ Falling
- ☐ Drooling or frothing
- ☐ Stiffening, jerking, or twitching of some muscles or the entire body
- ☐ Temporary loss of breathing with a red or blue face, followed by noisy respirations
- ☐ Loss of bowel or bladder control

How to prevent injury and choking during a seizure

1. Catch the person, if possible, when he falls, and lay him down. Someone with epilepsy may know when a convulsion is coming and may ask for your help.

2. Clear away furniture and all hard or sharp objects that may cause injury. Move the person only if he is near a fireplace, stairway, glass door, or other danger.

3. Loosen tight clothing around the person's neck and waist.

4. After the seizure stops, turn the person onto his side to prevent his choking on saliva, blood from a bitten tongue, or vomit.

5. Keep the person lying down. He will probably be too confused to walk safely. He will probably want to sleep. Let him. Don't be alarmed if there is loud snoring. Check carefully for injuries such as cuts and broken bones.

6. Seek medical attention if the person is not known to be epileptic or is pregnant, if the seizure does not stop within 2 minutes, or if another seizure begins shortly thereafter. Stay with the person until a medical professional is present.

What to do for seizures in children with high fever

1. Prevent injury and choking as in Steps 1-5 above.

2. Undress the child and reduce his fever by giving aspirin or acetaminophen and sponging with tepid water. This will help prevent another seizure. Do not place the child in a tub; if he has another seizure in the tub, he could inhale water.

3. Report the seizure to his doctor.

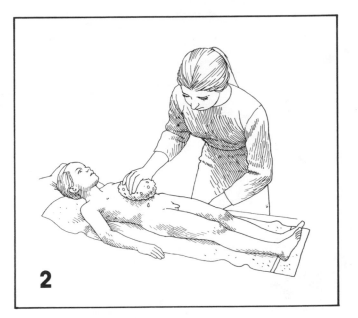

2

Ear Problems

overview:

There are five common ear emergencies including: swimmer's ear (caused by a fungus), ear pain (caused by infection, toothache, jaw joint pain), loss of hearing (caused by wax in the ear or perforation of the eardrum), drainage from the ear (most commonly caused by poking objects into the ear), and foreign bodies in the ear. All but foreign objects in the ear, **which you can see,** require immediate medical attention. Otherwise, loss of hearing and continued infection may result.

Water in the ear is not a medical emergency. You can treat it by putting a drop of rubbing alcohol into the ear. This lowers the surface tension of the water and provides relief.

Foreign objects in the ear can be removed in a few special instances, and insects in the ear can be killed. Usually, however, medical removal of the object or the insect is necessary.

98 Drainage from the ear

98 Foreign objects in the ear

Ear Problems

Drainage from the ear

Important—read first:

If bleeding from the ear follows a severe blow to the head (possible skull fracture), turn immediately to **Head Injuries,** page 120.

If bleeding is entirely from a cut on the outer ear, turn to **Bleeding,** page 37.

Do not put anything into the ear canal.

Do not try to stop drainage or bleeding from inside the ear.

Do not allow the person to thump his head to restore lost hearing.

Seek medical attention immediately.

Drainage from inside the ear (when there has been no serious head injury) may be due to a cut inside the ear or to a ruptured ear drum. Blood loss from inside the ear is never great, so the only major consideration is speedy medical care to determine and correct the cause. In the meantime, you can protect the ear from further damage as follows:

1. Cover the outside of the ear with a sterile or clean cloth pad, and bandage or tape it loosely in place.

2. Have the person lie on his side, with the affected ear down, to promote drainage.

Doctor's comments:

Bleeding from the ear after a severe blow to the head may be a sign of a skull fracture and should be treated accordingly.

Cuts inside the ear canal can be caused by foreign objects or by items poked into the ear, which may also rupture the eardrum. Other causes of ruptured eardrum include extremely loud noise, infection, a sudden change in air or water pressure (as in diving), or a blow to the ear. In most cases, the first-aider will be unable to distinguish between a ruptured eardrum and a cut, and must treat them the same.

Blood from inside the ear should be allowed to drain—not stopped—so that it does not back up through a ruptured eardrum and enter the deeper parts of the hearing mechanism.

Foreign objects in the ear

Important—read first:

Do not use any liquid to flush an object out of the ear.

Do not put any instrument into the ear canal.

Do not allow the person to thump his head to dislodge the object.

Flying or crawling insects occasionally become trapped in an ear; and children often put small objects, such as nuts, beads, or paper balls, into their ears, where they become lodged.

Stay calm. Although removal of the insect or object will usually require professional help, damage to the ear is rare.

Meanwhile, do the following:

A. If a live insect is trapped in the ear canal, you can kill it safely with a few drops of oil (mineral, olive, cooking, or baby oil). Let a doctor remove the dead insect.

OR

B. If paper, cotton, or cloth is in the ear and is clearly visible at the entrance to the ear canal, gently remove it with tweezers but do not reach inside the canal with the tweezers. A doctor should examine the ear to be sure that no material is left inside.

OR

C. If any other object (a bean, pea, bead, peanut, etc.) is trapped in the ear, the person should turn his head to the side—with the involved ear down—and shake his head. If this does not work, do not try anything else—no tweezers, water, oil, or hitting the head. Let a doctor remove the object.

Doctor's comments:

A live insect in the ear, especially if it is buzzing, can cause panic. Oil is safe in this case and will allow you to restore calm. With any other object, oil and water are dangerous because they may cause the object to swell, leading to pain and more difficult removal.

Trying to remove objects with tweezers can lead to a punctured eardrum. A doctor will have special instruments; he can use an otoscope to examine the eardrum and look for remaining foreign fragments.

Electric Shock

overview:

Electrical current follows the path of least resistance, usually the skin at low voltages, causing burns. However, damage to other tissues is possible, and high voltages can stop both breathing and heart action.

When a person has received an electric shock, first determine if he is still in contact with the current. If he is, shut it off if possible, or separate him from it while being careful not to be shocked yourself. Then call for medical assistance.

100 Rescue and first aid

Electric Shock
Rescue and first aid

Important—read first:

Remove the source of electricity before doing anything else.

Seek medical attention immediately for all electrical injuries and burns.

When you deal with electric shock, act quickly but remain calm and cautious so that you yourself do not become a victim.

First, separate the person from the source of electricity, then check his breathing, give CPR if necessary and if you are properly trained, and call for medical assistance.

Do not put butter or household remedies on burns or use pain-relief medication, ointment, or sprays without a doctor's instructions.

Do not press on a burned area or allow the person to walk on a burned foot.

Do not use cold water or ice on a large electrical burn (more than 2 inches across).

Do not open blisters or remove dead skin or clothing that sticks to a burned area.

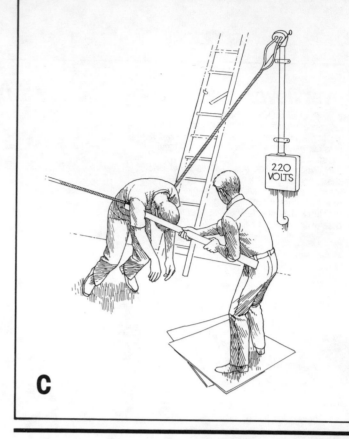

C

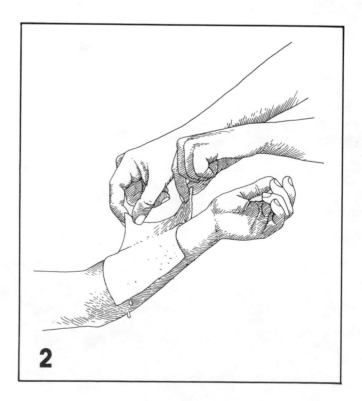

2

Doctor's comments:

To shut off electric current quickly and safely, don't waste time locating the correct small fuse or circuit breaker: Use the master cutoff in the fuse or circuit-breaker box. Flipping a wall switch or the switch on an appliance may turn off the appliance, but it will not remove the shock hazard, since only one of two wires is interrupted by a switch.

Electrical burns may appear minor, but they can extend deep into the tissue. All electrical burns are considered third-degree burns. Cold water should not be used if the burn is large because too-sudden cooling can increase the severity of shock.

Separate the person from the electricity

A. Do not expose yourself to the same hazard.

B. If the person is in contact with a wire or appliance, turn off the electric current by unplugging the wire or turning off the main circuit breaker or fuse for the entire house. Turning off an appliance or wall switch is not enough.

OR

C. If you cannot turn off the electricity, have someone else call the electric company. Stand on a dry insulating material such as thick newspaper or a rubber door mat. Use a dry, non-metallic (e.g., wooden) pole or board to push the person off the wire or the wire off the person.

D. If a person is near a live wire, keep him away from the electric hazard (e.g., if a car knocks down an electric pole, the person should stay inside the car) until help arrives.

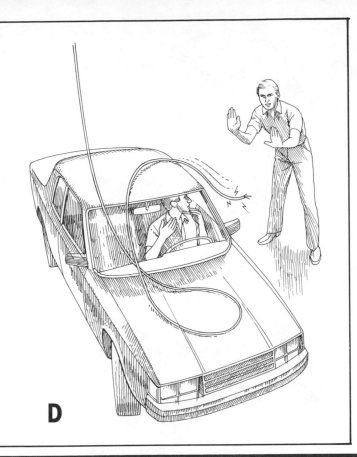

What to do while awaiting help

1. If you have time while waiting for the ambulance, look for two burns where electricity entered and exited the body.

2. Cover obviously burned areas with dressing.

Prevent shock

1. Seek medical attention as soon as possible. While awaiting the ambulance or while on the way to the emergency room, position the person as follows:

a. If the person is conscious, keep him lying on his back. Raise his legs 8 to 12 inches.

OR

b. If he is unconscious, place him on his side, with his head supported by his arm or a pillow. Bend his top knee to keep him from rolling forward.

2. Cover him lightly with a blanket or jacket. If he is on a cold surface, place a blanket underneath him as well.

For details on rescue from electric shock read the manual on this subject provided by your local electric company.

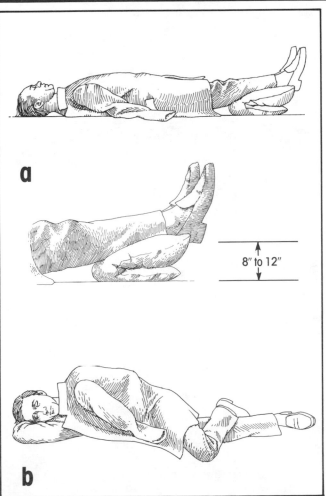

8" to 12"

101

Eye Injuries

overview:

Injuries involving the globe (eyeball) are potentially dangerous, and require medical attention, **especially** if there is a **change in vision.**

Foreign objects that are resting on the eyeball or on the inside of the eyelid can be washed out, but foreign objects that are embedded in the eye or that do not wash out must be treated by a doctor.

For a chemical burn of the eye, flush the eye immediately and copiously and seek medical attention.

104-105 Loose or invisible objects in the eye

106 Object embedded in the eye

107 Chemical burns of the eye

108 Cuts & blunt injuries (black eye)

Eye Injuries
Loose or invisible object in the eye

Important—read first:

Do not allow the person to rub or press on the eye.

Do not try to remove contact lenses.

If an object you thought was loose does not wash out, cover both eyes and seek medical attention immediately.

Seek medical attention promptly if pain, tearing, or blurred vision continues after a loose object has been removed.

Signs of a foreign body in the eye

- ☐ Stinging or burning pain, especially when blinking
- ☐ Redness or "bloodshot" appearance
- ☐ Tearing
- ☐ Sensitivity to light

If any of these signs are present, wash your hands thoroughly with soap and water then examine the eye in good light.

If you see a foreign object sticking into the eyeball, follow instructions under **Object embedded in the eye,** on page 106.

If a cinder, speck, or eyelash seems to be resting on the surface of the eyeball or on the inner surface of the eyelid, or if you cannot see the object, follow instructions at right.

Doctor's comments:
   If irritation or other symptoms continue after a loose foreign object has been removed from the eye, the object may have scratched the cornea (the clear covering of the pupil). An ophthalmologist or emergency room doctor can quickly check for corneal injury, which usually heals in 24-48 hours when covered with an eye patch.

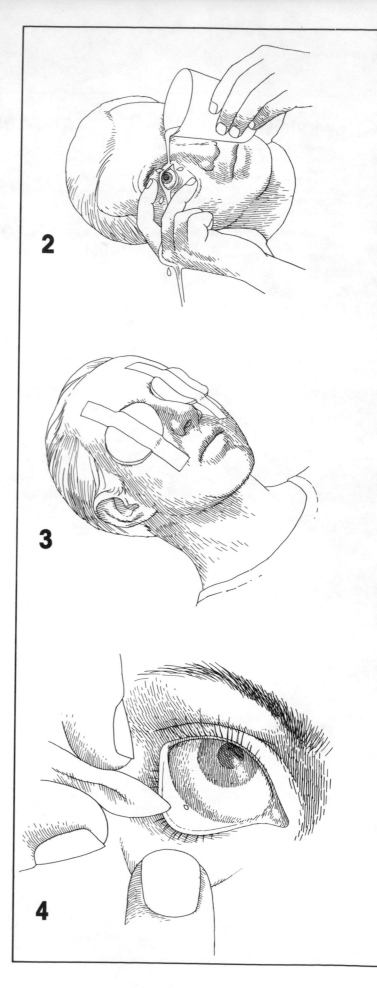

2

3

4

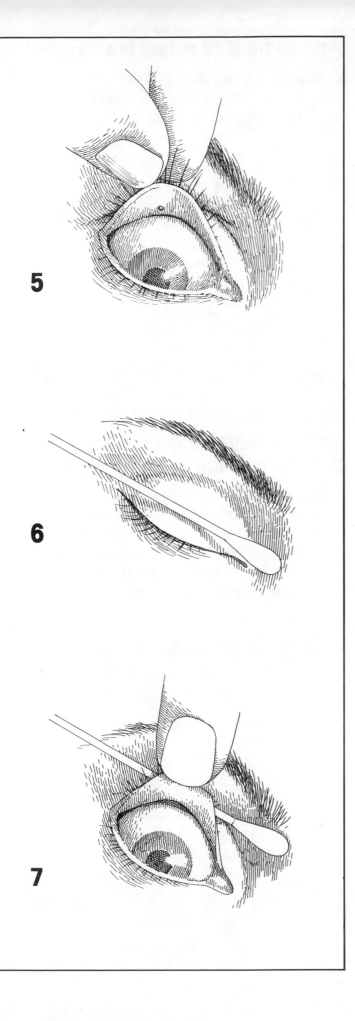

5

6

7

First, try to flush the object out

1. Tearing by itself may flush the object free.

2. If tearing does not work, gently flush the eye with lukewarm water squeezed from an eyedropper or poured from a glass.

If flushing does not remove an object you can see, treat as for an embedded object

3. Cover both eyes with sterile or clean cloth pads, bandage or tape them loosely in place, and seek medical assistance.

If flushing does not work and you cannot see the object, look for it

4. Gently pull the lower lid down and look at its inner surface while the person looks up. If you see a particle, gently flush the eye with lukewarm water, as above.

5. If no object is visible inside the lower lid, check the upper lid. If you see a particle on the inner surface of the upper lid, you can turn the lid over to get at it.

6. Tell the person to look down during this entire procedure. Pull gently downward on the upper eyelashes. Lay a swab or matchstick across the top of the lid.

7. Fold the lid up over the swab or matchstick. Gently flush the eye with lukewarm water, as above. Then gently pull the upper lid back down by the lashes.

If irritation continues, cover the eyes

8. If pain, tearing, or blurred vision continues after the foreign object has been removed, or if symptoms continue despite the fact that you never find the object, seek medical attention. These symptoms may be the result of a scratch on the surface of the eye (cornea).

Eye Injuries
Object embedded in the eye

Important—read first:

Do not remove an embedded object.

Do not allow the person to rub or press on the eye.

Do not try to remove contact lenses.

Seek medical attention immediately.

Signs of a foreign body in the eye

- ☐ History of the event
- ☐ Stinging or burning pain, especially when blinking
- ☐ Redness or "bloodshot" appearance
- ☐ Tearing
- ☐ Sensitivity to light (photophobia)

If any of these signs are present, wash your hands thoroughly with soap and water, then examine the eye in good light.

If a cinder, speck, or eyelash seems to be resting on the surface of the eyeball or on the inner surface of the eyelid, or if you cannot see the object, follow instructions under **Loose or invisible object** on page 105.

If you see an object sticking into the eyeball, do the following:

If an embedded object is small

A. Have the person close his eyes. Cover both eyes with sterile or clean cloth pads, and bandage or tape them loosely in place.

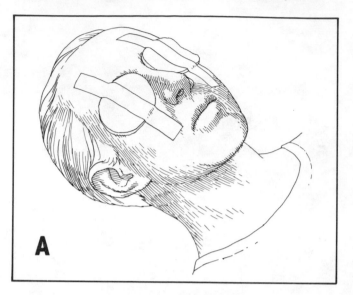

A

If an embedded object is large and prevents the eye from closing

B. Take a paper cup or make a paper cone large enough to cover the embedded object without touching it. Set the cup or cone over the eye, and tape it securely in place. Cover the other eye with a clean cloth pad, and tape or bandage it loosely in place.

For all embedded objects

C. Keep the person flat on his back while on the way to the nearest emergency room.

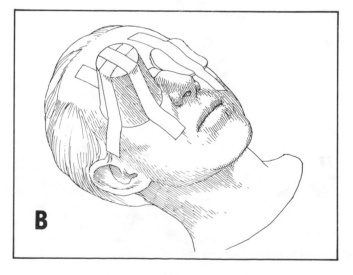

B

Doctor's comments:

When an object is embedded in the eye, any pressure can cause further damage. For this reason, a bandage or tape over the eye must be loose; and pressing, rubbing, and contact lens removal must be avoided. Since the eyes move together, when one eye is injured, both must be covered to prevent movement of the injured eye.

Eye Injuries
Chemical burns of the eye

Important—read first:

Flush the eye immediately and thoroughly, then seek medical attention at once.

Do not contaminate the uninjured eye.

Do not allow the person to rub his eye.

Do not try to remove contact lenses.

When chemicals or household products get into the eye, immediate and copious washing can prevent blindness.

1. Turn the person's head to the side, keeping the uninjured eye higher so that the chemical does not get into it. Hold the injured eye wide open with your fingers and flush with large amounts of cool water, washing the entire eye from its inside corner (near the nose) outward. The water may be from a faucet, a drinking fountain, or a container. Use milk if you have no water. **Continue to flush for 10 full minutes.**

2. Cover both eyes with sterile or clean cloth pads, and bandage or tape them loosely in place.

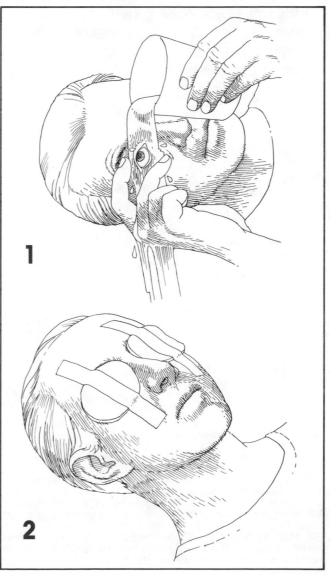

Doctor's comments:

Any solid, liquid, or gaseous chemicals, including acids, alkalies, household cleaning and bleaching products, and many weaker chemicals that would not burn the skin, can damage the delicate tissues of the eye. Thorough flushing and prompt transportation to an emergency room are advisable if there is any doubt about the safety of a product that has gotten into the eye.

Attempts to neutralize the chemical may be harmful and are sure to waste precious time.

Since the eyes move together, when one eye is injured, both must be covered to prevent movement of the injured eye.

Eye Injuries
Cuts & blunt injuries (black eye)

Important—read first:

Seek medical attention immediately for all cuts or blunt injuries to the eye or the area of the cheek or forehead immediately surrounding the eye.

Do not try to remove contact lenses.

Do not allow the person to rub his eye.

Do not press on the eye to control bleeding.

Do not wash the eye.

If someone has been struck on or around the eye, check to see if there has also been a cut and a loss of vision which is the common denominator for serious eye injury.

Cuts on the eye

Treat all cuts on the eyeball, on the lids, and around the eye as potentially very serious.

1. Cover both eyes with sterile or clean cloth pads, and bandage or tape them loosely in place.

2. Keep the person in a semi-reclining position while on the way to an ophthalmologist or the nearest emergency room.

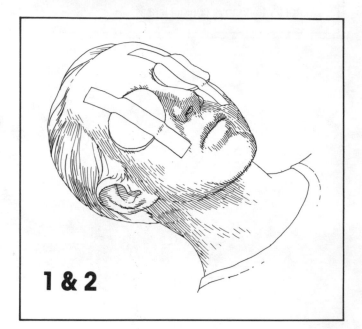

1 & 2

Blunt injuries (including a black eye)

A blunt injury to the eye by a fist, ball, or other object may be more serious than it appears. To be on the safe side, do the following:

1. Have the person lie on his back with his eyes closed.

2. Place a folded cloth soaked in cold water gently on the eye.

3. Seek medical attention.

Doctor's comments:
To prevent further damage to a cut eye, all pressure on the eye must be avoided. For this reason, a bandage or tape must be loose, and pressure should not be used to control bleeding from the lid or eye, which is never serious enough to be life-threatening. Rubbing or washing the eye, applying a wet compress, or trying to remove contact lenses also could cause dangerous pressure.

Since the eyes move together, when one eye is injured, both must be covered to prevent movement of the injured eye.

Cuts on the eyelid are not dangerous in themselves, but they sometimes involve cuts of the eyeball that may not be obvious, especially if the lid is bleeding into the eye.

Although a "black eye" is usually not serious, blunt injuries sometimes can cause immediate or delayed bleeding inside the eye or cause a contact lens to cut the eye's surface. A professional eye examination may be needed to detect these conditions.

Exposure
to Heat & Cold

overview:

Prolonged exposure to high temperature can cause heatstroke (sunstroke) or heat exhaustion. Heatstroke requires rapid cooling to lower dangerously high body temperature. Heatstroke is a life-threatening condition.

Hypothermia is lowered overall body temperature caused either by low temperatures, dampness and cool winds, or prolonged exposure to water. Significant hypothermia does not require freezing temperatures, particularly in elderly persons who are at risk at temperatures higher than 32°F. Warm the person with dry clothing and blankets and seek medical attention immediately. Prolonged exposure to cold can cause a life threatening lowering of body temperature with or without frostbite.

Frostbite is freezing of the tissue. The frostbitten part should be rewarmed. If a part of the body is frostbitten, reheat it quickly in warm water and elevate the part, and have the person exercise it on the way to an Emergency Room. All frostbite injuries should be seen in an Emergency Room. Proper rewarming of a frostbitten part is only the first stage in treatment. Judging the severity of frostbite after rewarming may be difficult and requires trained medical personnel, as does tetanus prophylaxis, for proper after-care and rehabilitation.

110-111 Heatstroke (sunstroke) & heat exhaustion

112 Hypothermia (lowered body temperature)

113 Frostbite

Exposure to Heat & Cold

Heatstroke (sunstroke) & heat exhaustion

Important—read first:

Do not give the person beverages with alcohol or caffeine (coffee, tea, or certain sodas—check the label).

For heatstroke, seek medical attention immediately.

For heat exhaustion, seek medical attention immediately after cooling the person if symptoms are prolonged, or worsen despite treatment, or include vomiting, fainting, or convulsions.

Heatstroke and heat exhaustion are treated differently. Heatstroke is a medical emergency and requires immediate medical attention and transportation to a hospital. Read the signs for heatstroke and heat exhaustion and treat whichever condition is present. If in doubt, treat for heatstroke.

Signs of heatstroke

☐ Body temperature 102°F or higher
☐ Skin red and hot
☐ No sweating
☐ Confusion or unconsciousness
☐ Fainting
☐ Convulsions

First aid for heatstroke

1. Move the person to a cool place. Seek medical attention immediately. Spray the person with a hose, sponge him with cold water or alcohol, or throw a pail of water on him while massaging the extremities and torso.

2. Check the person's temperature every 10 minutes. When his temperature is below 102°F, dry him off; but if it rises again above 102°F, repeat the cooling procedure.

3. Keep the person cool with an air conditioner or fan while awaiting help or while on the way to the nearest emergency room.

Doctor's comments:

Heatstroke (also called sunstroke) occurs when extremely high temperatures overwhelm the body's heat-control system. Fevers as high as 108°F have occurred with heatstroke, and such high internal temperatures can cause brain damage or even death. Alcoholic beverages and stimulants such as caffeine can add to the body's inability to regulate heat.

Heat exhaustion is caused by the loss of salt and fluid during heavy sweating, and by the body's attempts to cool itself by directing so much blood to the skin that circulation to internal organs is impaired. Drinking saltwater and lying down with legs raised help correct the fluid and salt deficits and increase blood flow to the brain and organs of the torso. When people exercise strenuously on hot, humid days, heat exhaustion often begins with "heat cramps," especially in the muscles of the abdomen and legs.

Medically defined, the core temperature for heatstroke is 105°. However, a temperature of 102° or higher when combined with any of the other symptoms listed above should be taken as an alert to the possibility of a problem that requires medical attention.

Signs of heat exhaustion

- Body temperature above 98.6°F but below 102°F
- Skin pale and clammy
- Heavy sweating
- Dizziness or fainting
- Tiredness and weakness
- Nausea and vomiting
- Headache
- Muscle cramps

First aid for heat exhaustion

1. Move the person to a cool place—an air-conditioned room or car, a cool room, or the shade. Have him lie on his back with his legs elevated 8 to 12 inches.

2. Loosen his clothing, and cool him gently with wet cloths or a fan if there is no air conditioning.

3. Add 1 teaspoon of salt to a quart of cool water and have the person sip it slowly over half an hour. Repeat with a second glass. Stop giving liquid if the person vomits. Flat soda pop or similar nonalcoholic beverages also can be given.

4. If heat cramps occur, massage the cramped muscles firmly until they relax.

5. Seek medical help immediately if symptoms continue for more than an hour, if they worsen during treatment, or if they include muscle cramps, vomiting, fainting, or convulsions.

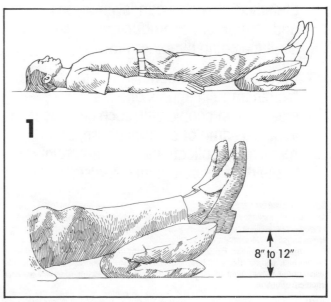

8" to 12"

Exposure to Heat & Cold
Hypothermia
(lowered body temperature)

Important—read first:

If the person registers a temperature on a regular thermometer and is shivering, he probably does not have significant hypothermia. Simply move the person to a warm place, remove any wet or damp clothing and warm him.

Significant hypothermia is suspected immediately when a person has a temperature too low to register on a normal thermometer. Seek medical attention immediately.

Do not assume that a "lifeless" person found in the cold is dead. He may be deeply unconscious, with very faint pulse and breathing.

When taking temperature for hypothermia, be sure to shake the mercury in the thermometer way down. (For instructions on how to take a temperature, see **Fever,** page 117.

Do not warm the person rapidly with hot water or a heat lamp.

Do not give the person alcoholic beverages.

After wrapping the person warmly, seek medical attention immediately.

Prolonged exposure to cold outdoor temperatures, cold water, or underheated rooms can lower overall body temperature, producing life-threatening hypothermia.

Even less extreme conditions can produce hypothermia in infants and the elderly, or in people with such complicating factors as drug or alcohol abuse, or medical complications such as cardiovascular or neurological disorders.

Doctor's comments:
Even in not very low temperatures, total body cooling can occur with prolonged exposure if the person is poorly dressed or inadequately nourished, or if high winds cause a severe wind-chill factor.

Those at high risk for developing hypothermia include infants, the elderly, people with chronic heart or lung problems, very thin individuals, and people who cannot move about to keep warm because of paralysis, arthritis, or other medical conditions.

Signs of hypothermia

- ☐ Exposure to cold outdoor temperatures, cold water, or underheated rooms
- ☐ No longer shivering and "feeling cold" (both may stop when body temperature falls below 90°F)
- ☐ Drowsiness and weakness
- ☐ Skin pale, bluish, bright pink, or puffy
- ☐ Slurred speech and confusion
- ☐ Unconsciousness and rigid muscles

Additional signs of hypothermia in infants

- ☐ Red cheeks, chin, tip of the nose or limbs
- ☐ No crying
- ☐ Weak sucking when fed

If any of these signs are present in a person exposed to the cold, do the following:

1. Take the person to a warm room, if possible.

2. Remove any wet clothing, and wrap the person in blankets, towels, clothing, or other heavy insulation. An additional outer layer of aluminum foil is helpful and easy to apply with infants. Body warmth may also help.

3. If the person is conscious, give him any warm, nonalcoholic drink.

4. Seek medical attention.

Exposure to Heat & Cold
Frostbite

Extremely cold temperatures can freeze parts of the body that are exposed or have poor circulation, especially fingers, toes, the nose, and the ears. This is made worse by wet gloves or clothing and by high winds. As the frozen tissue is rewarmed, it may swell, blister, and become discolored. This will require proper and prompt medical attention.

Signs of frostbite

- ☐ Skin red and painful (early in frostbite)
- ☐ Skin turns white or mottled, firm, waxy, and numb (with deeper freezing)
- ☐ Blisters

If any of these signs are present, do the following:

1. Place the frostbitten part(s) inside the person's clothing, next to his body for warmth, or wrap with clothing or a scarf then get the person indoors quickly.

2. Put the frostbitten part(s) in warm (not hot) water. Measure the water temperature with a thermometer. The water temperature should be 104-108 degrees F (40-42 degrees C). If you have no warm water, keep the part(s) wrapped warmly. Remove any rings or other constricting jewelry or clothing.

3. After the frostbitten part becomes pink and numbness begins to fade, stop the rewarming. Put sterile or clean gauze or cloth over any broken blisters and between frostbitten fingers and toes.

4. Seek medical care immediately. While waiting for the ambulance or while on the way to the nearest emergency room, keep the frostbitten part wrapped to prevent refreezing.

Doctor's comments:

Rewarming should be prompt but gentle. Rubbing may damage the frozen skin. Fires, stoves, and other sources of high heat can cause burns while the skin is still numb.

Alcohol and tobacco must be avoided. Alcohol interferes with the body's heat-regulating system, and tobacco decreases blood circulation in the skin.

Refreezing of the same part after it has been warmed is extremely dangerous. If the part cannot be kept warm while you are seeking medical care, it is less damaging to leave the part frozen than to warm it and have it freeze again.

Fever
Fever and Rashes

overview:

Fever is the result of the body's response to infection or inflammation and is the body's primary symptom of illness. If you suspect fever, take the person's temperature. A high fever (greater than 102 degrees F) is usually a reason to contact your physician or seek medical attention. Reducing fever by first-aid methods does not correct the underlying problem.

116-117 General treatment

118 Fever & rashes

Fever

Important—read first:

Do not use rubbing alcohol, cold baths, ice packs, enemas, or alcoholic beverages to treat fever.

Do not give any medication to someone with a fever caused by heatstroke (sunstroke). To treat heatstroke, see **Exposure to Heat & Cold,** page 110.

Consult a doctor for:

☐ Any fever in a child
☐ A fever of 102°F (38.9°C) in an adult
☐ A sudden rise in temperature
☐ Fever lasting more than one day with no other symptoms to suggest a common cause

Seek medical attention immediately for:

☐ Convulsions caused by fever (see **Convulsions,** page 94)
☐ Fever with pain when the person tries to bend his neck (possible meningitis)

In most instances, fever is part of the body's natural reaction to mild infection.
The purpose of first aid is primarily to ease discomfort and prevent dehydration. It also lessens the chance of convulsions in young children.

Doctor's comments:

Normal temperature varies slightly from person to person. It changes with exercise and even with the time of day (lower in the morning, higher in the evening). Rectal temperature is about 1 degree Fahrenheit higher than oral temperature.

Fever is usually a sign of infection, especially if it begins suddenly with chills. The use of medication for mild fever is currently a topic of debate. Seen as the body's effective defense mechanism against infection, fever may shorten an illness, increase the power of antibiotics, and make an infection less contagious. These possible advantages must be weighed against the discomfort involved in letting a slight fever run its course.

It is, however, important to reduce very high fever. In children under 6 years old, temperatures of 102°F (orally) or higher can trigger convulsions. Adults, especially those with chronic illnesses (heart or respiratory diseases), may not be able to tolerate prolonged high body temperature.

It is also important to follow directions precisely when giving any medication, even the mild, safe nonprescription medicines used for fever. Both aspirin and acetaminophen can result in harmful overdoses if given improperly. Aspirin should be stopped if it causes stomach irritation (or hyperventilation, especially in children), and it should not be used by people with bleeding disorders or those taking certain other medications. Discuss fever medications with your doctor.

Some traditional treatments for fever are dangerous and should not be used. These include ice packs, cold baths, and cold enemas, all of which can cause shock through overly rapid cooling. Alcohol in drinks interferes with the body's heat-control mechanism. Alcohol used in sponge baths given to babies can be absorbed through the skin or inhaled as it evaporates, with serious consequences.

Fever—General treatment

1. Take the person's temperature. Use a rectal thermometer for small children, people with mouth injuries, and people who cannot breathe through their noses (they'll be unable to keep their mouths closed). For anyone else, you may use either an oral or a rectal thermometer. Do not take oral temperature for at least a half hour after the person has had hot or cold food or drink or has smoked; altered mouth temperatures will give a falsely high or low reading. Within a half hour after exercise or a hot bath, oral and rectal temperature will be falsely high as well. If you are unsure about the use of a thermometer, see instructions on opposite page.

2. If temperature is elevated, remove excess clothing or covers from the person, leaving just enough so that he is not chilly.

3. Encourage the person to rest and to drink plenty of fluids—any type he prefers except alcoholic beverages.

4. Medications containing aspirin (Bufferin®, Anacin®, etc.) or acetaminophen (Tylenol®, Anacin II®, etc.) help reduce fever and some symptoms that often accompany it. Each has certain advantages and disadvantages depending on the individual and the situation. Ask your doctor which is best for each member of your family. Always check with a doctor, if possible, before giving any medication to a young child, especially an infant under 1 year old. When you give these medications, follow the directions or package instructions exactly.

Very high fever—additional treatment

1. For high fever (102°F/38.9°C orally; 103°F/39.4C° rectally), consult your doctor and bring the temperature down with a sponge bath: Sit the person in a tub with 6–10 inches of tepid or lukewarm water so that most of his body is exposed to the air.
OR

2. If no tub is available, place a towel under the person in bed and bring water to the bedside in a basin or pail. Briskly wipe water onto his entire body with a sponge or a washcloth (or scoop and spread water over him with your hand). Let it evaporate from his skin. Avoid drafts, and stop if the person develops chills.

3. Continue for 20 to 30 minutes, then check his temperature. If it is still over 101° F/38.3°C orally or 102°F/38.9°C rectally, continue the sponge bath for another 15 minutes and check again. If fever remains high, consult your doctor again.

4. Briskly rub the person dry with a towel.

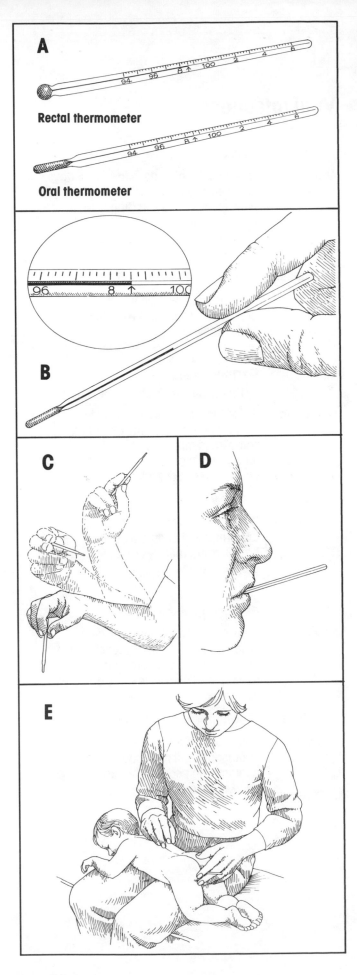

Rectal thermometer

Oral thermometer

Using a thermometer oral and rectal

If you aren't sure how to use an oral or a rectal thermometer, here are the basics. Knowing the proper technique is especially important when taking an infant's temperature.

A. **Types of thermometers.** An oral thermometer has a long, thin metal bulb at the end for faster heating. A rectal thermometer has a short, fat bulb, so it is less sharp. If necessary, an oral thermometer can be used—very gently—to take a rectal temperature, and a rectal thermometer sterilized with alcohol (or a brand-new one) can be used in the mouth.

B. **How to read.** All thermometers have a thin red or silver column of mercury in the center. Hold one end between your thumb and forefinger, the numbers and lines facing you. Rotate it slightly until you can see the red or silver column. The tip of the mercury column indicates the temperature. Each degree is marked by a line, with shorter lines in between marking each two-tenths of a degree. Usually, only even-degree lines are numbered (because of a lack of space). An **arrow** usually points to 98.6°F/37°C—normal oral temperature (even if it's a rectal thermometer!).

C. **First, shake it down.** Before taking anyone's temperature, shake the thermometer until the mercury column is well below 98.6°F/37°C. Hold the end opposite the bulb and use sharp, snapping wrist movements. If you do this over a bed, the thermometer won't break if you drop it.

D. **To take an oral temperature:** Place the bulb of the thermometer under the tongue. Tell the person to keep his lips closed, and warn him not to talk or bite. Leave the thermometer in for 3 full minutes before reading.

E. **To take a baby's rectal temperature:** Sit down and lay the baby face-down on your lap. (To take an older person's rectal temperature, have him lie on his stomach.) Dip the bulb in Vaseline or cold cream. Separate the buttocks, and insert the bulb gently about 1 inch into the rectum. Never use force; if the thermometer meets resistance, gently change the angle until it slips in easily. Let go of the thermometer and place your hand across the baby's buttocks, with the thermometer held lightly between two fingers. Leave it in for 3 full minutes and wipe with a tissue before reading.

Fever
Fever & rashes

Important—read first:

Do not use rubbing alcohol, cold baths, ice packs, enemas, or alcoholic beverages to treat fever.

Do not give any medication to someone with a fever caused by heatstroke (sunstroke). To treat heatstroke, see **Exposure to Heat & Cold,** page 110.

Consult a doctor for:

☐ Any fever in a child
☐ A fever of 102°F (38.9°C) in an adult
☐ A sudden rise in temperature
☐ Fever lasting more than one day with no other symptoms to suggest a common cause

Seek medical attention immediately for:

☐ Convulsions caused by fever (see **Convulsions,** page 94)
☐ Fever with pain when the person tries to bend his neck (possible meningitis)

Doctor's comments:

Normal temperature varies slightly from person to person. It changes with exercise and even with the time of day (lower in the morning, higher in the evening). Rectal temperature is about 1 degree Fahrenheit higher than oral temperature.

Fever is usually a sign of infection, especially if it begins suddenly with chills.

The use of medication for mild fever is currently a topic of debate. Seen as the body's effective defense mechanism against infection, fever may shorten an illness, increase the power of antibiotics, and make an infection less contagious. These possible advantages must be weighed against the discomfort involved in letting a slight fever run its course.

It is, however, important to reduce very high fever. In children under 6 years old, temperatures of 102°F (orally) or higher can trigger convulsions. Adults, especially those with chronic illnesses (heart or respiratory diseases), may not be able to tolerate prolonged high body temperature.

It is also important to follow directions precisely when giving any medication, even the mild, safe nonprescription medicines used for fever. Both aspirin and acetaminophen can result in harmful overdoses if given improperly. Aspirin should be stopped if it causes stomach irritation (or hyperventilation, especially in children), and it should not be used by people with bleeding disorders or those taking certain other medications. Discuss fever medications with your doctor.

Some traditional treatments for fever are dangerous and should not be used. These include ice packs, cold baths, and cold enemas, all of which can cause shock through overly rapid cooling. Alcohol in drinks interferes with the body's heat-control mechanism. Alcohol used in sponge baths given to babies can be absorbed through the skin or inhaled as it evaporates, with serious consequences.

Viral infections

Measles

Appearance: fever and running nose for 3 or 4 days, followed by the eruption of flat, pink spots, usually starting near the ears and spreading. Look for tiny, red-ringed white spots on the roof of the mouth.

Cause: rubeola virus

First aid: Call a doctor. Avoid contact with unimmunized people who have not had measles.

German measles ("three-day measles," rubella)

Appearance: flat or raised pink spots, usually starting on the face and spreading; sometimes mildly itchy. Look for swollen glands behind the ears and on the sides and back of the neck.

Cause: rubella virus

First aid: Call a doctor. Avoid contact with unimmunized people who have not had German measles and with pregnant women.

Chicken pox

Appearance: fever for 1 day, followed by the eruption of red pimples that change to blisters, break, and form crusts; usually starting on the body and always very itchy.

Cause: varicella virus

First aid: Call a doctor. Avoid the spread of pus to other parts of the body. Avoid contact with people who have not had chicken pox.

Head Injuries

overview:

First aid for skull and scalp injuries has three goals: (1) recognizing the signs of skull fractures and concussions, (2) positioning the person to prevent shock, and (3) controlling bleeding, which may be profuse, from scalp wounds.

**120 Skull & scalp
(including forehead)**

Head Injuries
Skull & scalp
(including forehead)

Important—read first:

Check for neck injuries after any serious blow to the head. If the person is conscious, ask if he is aware of pain in the neck, paralysis, weakness, numbness or tingling of an arm or leg; if the person is unconscious and a pinprick to each palm does not cause a reflex movement, suspect a neck injury. Immobilize the head and neck as described in **Back & Neck Injuries,** page 17.

Do not move the person more than is absolutely necessary.

Do not clean severe head wounds or remove embedded material.

Do not remove impaled objects.

Do not attempt to arouse the person with stimulants such as smelling salts.

Note the time of any head injury and the time at which the person loses and regains consciousness.

Do not give anything to eat or drink.

Seek medical assistance immediately.

Signs of possible severe head injury requiring medical attention

Signs of a possible skull fracture or concussion may appear immediately after an accident or at any time over a 48-hour period. They include:

☐ Unconsciousness, drowsiness, or disorientation
☐ A depression in the scalp
☐ Blood or clear fluid coming from the nose, ear, or mouth (do not try to stop the flow)
☐ Bruising around an eye or behind an ear
☐ Paralysis of one side of the body
☐ Loss of vision
☐ Convulsions
☐ Vomiting
☐ Slurred speech
☐ Loss of memory for or around event
☐ Persistent or severe headaches

If none of these signs is present and the person has only a minor cut, turn to **Bleeding,** page 37, and treat as instructed.

If any of the above signs appears after a blow or injury to the head, or if there is a serious cut in the scalp or forehead, give first aid as described at right and seek medical attention.

Doctor's comments:
  Skull fractures, particularly if they are depressed (dented in), may result in brain injury, but many skull fractures cause no brain damage at all. On the other hand, a blow to the head or even sudden stopping of the head's motion (as in a car accident) may not cause a fracture but may cause the brain to strike the inside of the skull, producing concussion or other brain injury. Most concussions clear quickly and leave the person with no impairment.
  Skull fractures may cause internal bleeding or allow clear cerebrospinal fluid to leak out. The only signs of skull fracture may be fluid or blood in the ear or nose, or under the skin, where it appears as a discoloration around the eyes (a "raccoon sign") or behind the ear.
  Cuts on the scalp commonly result from falls and blunt injuries, when the skin and muscle of the scalp are pressed forcefully against the hard skull and cut from within. These scalp wounds tend to be deep and to bleed freely. Cleaning the wound can make the bleeding worse. If an underlying fracture is remotely possible, contamination of the skull (and brain) must be avoided, so cleaning should take place in the emergency room, not at the scene of the injury.
  The time at which a head injury occurs and at which a person loses and regains consciousness should be noted so that medical personnel can calculate the length of unconsciousness and how soon it followed the injury.
  Food and drink should be avoided, as vomiting often occurs after even minor head injuries.
  A person who has suffered any sort of head injury should be observed for 48 hours in the event that danger signs develop. On the first night after a head injury, check the person every 3 hours or so to see that he can be awakened.

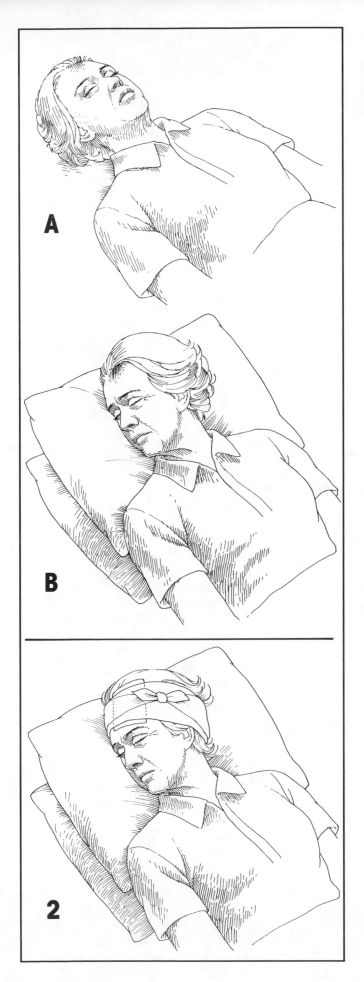

First aid for skull and scalp injuries, possible fracture, concussion, or serious cut

1. Keep the person lying down. Use one of two positions:

A. If the person is unconscious, or his face is pale, or there are any signs of neck injury, keep his head on the same level as his body.

OR

B. If he is conscious and the color of his face is normal or red, and there are no signs of neck injury, raise his head and shoulders (not just his head) slightly by placing on a pillow or some other soft object. Turn his head gently to one side to avoid choking if he vomits.

2. If the scalp is cut, control bleeding while awaiting help or while on the way to an emergency room. Cover the wound completely with a sterile or clean cloth pad, and press firmly but gently over the entire wound.

3. Keep the person comfortably warm. Call for medical assistance. If you must transport him to an emergency room, have him lie in whichever of the two positions is applicable (1A or 1B). If, however, there are any signs of a neck injury, do not transport the person; immobilize the head and neck. See **Back & Neck Injuries, page 17.**

Heart Attack &
Chest Pain

overview:

When chest pain occurs, check the list of danger signs to see if a heart problem is likely. If it is, have the person sit or lie semi-reclined, loosen clothing around his neck, try to calm him, and seek medical assistance immediately. If the person has medication for angina, help him take it.

Turn immediately to p. 124.

Heart Attack & Chest Pain

Important—read first:

If you are properly trained, be ready to use CPR if breathing stops.

Do not let the person exert himself.

Seek medical attention immediately.

Chest pain may be caused by lung or muscle problems that are not emergencies.

But if the pain resembles the description at right or is accompanied by any of the other danger signs listed, be safe by assuming that it is a heart attack or angina.

Seek medical care, and follow the first aid instructions on the opposite page while waiting for the ambulance or while on the way to the nearest emergency room.

Signs of a possible heart attack (or of angina pectoris)

☐ Pain
- lasting more than 2 minutes
- usually described as "tight" or "crushing"
- usually in the center of the chest
- sometimes spreading to the upper abdomen, shoulder or arm (usually the left), neck, or jaw

☐ Gasping or shortness of breath that improves when the person rests or sits (but gets worse when he lies flat)

☐ Severe anxiety—feeling of impending doom

☐ Weakness

☐ Heavy sweating, even without exercise

☐ Pale or bluish skin or lips

☐ Nausea or vomiting

☐ Irregular pulse

Doctor's comments:

Most chest pains do not involve the heart, so reassurance is appropriate. Pain in the chest may be caused by indigestion, strained muscles, lung infections, shingles (a virus-caused condition involving the nerves of the skin), and numerous other nonemergencies.

The vice-like squeezing symptoms of true heart pain occur when not enough blood and oxygen can reach the heart muscle. This can result in:

• **Angina pectoris**—temporary pain, usually followed by complete recovery. It is caused by temporary spasm of the heart's own blood vessels (the coronary arteries) or by overexertion in someone with narrowed coronary arteries. A nitroglycerine pill under the tongue or the inhaling of amyl nitrate, together with rest, usually provides relief within 5 minutes. Do not give these medications to a person unless he has had some prescribed specifically for him. (NOTE: If an angina patient's nitroglycerine pill does not work, ask him if it stings his tongue. It should. If it doesn't, it is old and has lost its potency. The person should not panic).

• **Heart attack** (also "myocardial infarction" or "coronary thrombosis")—prolonged pain with destruction of a piece of heart muscle. It is caused by completely closed coronary artery. Heart attacks often occur when the person is at rest, hours after strenuous exercise. The person should get to the nearest emergency room as quickly as possible.

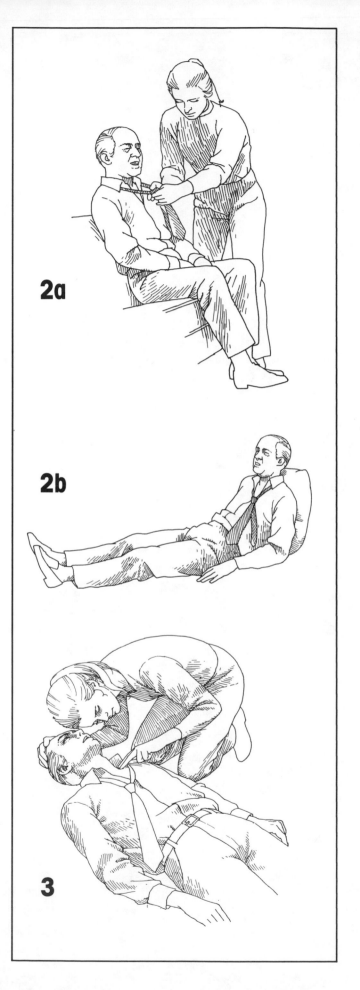

2a

2b

3

First aid for heart attack or angina

1. Your first priority is to contact medical help. Call 911 or an emergency medical team as soon as possible.

2. Have the person (a) sit up or (b) lie semi-reclined (let him choose the more comfortable of the two positions). Loosen clothing, such as a tight collar or necktie, around his neck. Keep him comfortably warm if the air is chilly. Calm him as much as possible.

3. If the person loses consciousness, lay him flat on his back and check for breathing and pulse. If he vomits, turn his head to the side and clean his mouth.

4. If the person has medicine for angina pectoris and is conscious, help him take it. Prompt relief of chest pain means that this is probably another angina attack (temporary shortage of oxygen to the heart), not a heart attack (serious and sustained shortage of oxygen to the heart).

5. If breathing stops, and you are trained in CPR, give cardiopulmonary resuscitation.

Mouth Injuries

overview:

Bleeding inside the mouth can be controlled with direct pressure, using different techniques for different parts of the mouth.

128 Bleeding in the mouth

Mouth Injuries
Bleeding in the mouth

Important—read first:

If a serious face injury or broken jaw is suspected, turn immediately to page 90.

Minor accidents frequently cause bleeding from one or more parts of the mouth. Bleeding will often look more severe than it really is, so stay calm, reassure the injured person, and follow instructions at right.

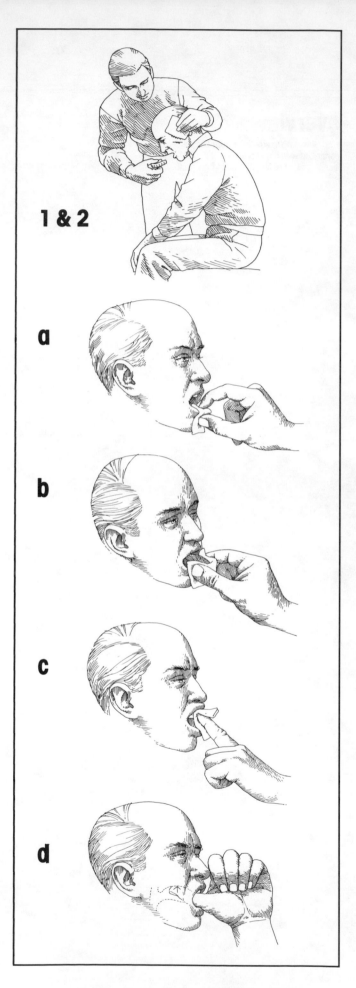

1 & 2

a

b

c

d

Doctor's comments:

  Most cuts in the mouth are caused by relatively clean objects, such as utensils, toothbrushes, fists, and the person's own teeth. But if a dirty object strikes the mouth, or if the lip is cut in a fall against the ground, a tetanus booster is advisable if none has been received within 10 years.

  When pressing on the roof of the mouth to stop bleeding, the injured person's own thumb is less likely to cause gagging than is someone else's thumb.

  Used tea bags are excellent for dental bleeding because the tannic acid in them helps constrict blood vessels and promote clotting in the tooth socket. Reimplantations of unbroken teeth have become fairly routine. They are usually successful if done quickly. In general, there is about a 50 percent chance of a reimplant "taking" at 1½ hours. Some reimplants have worked even when performed a day or more after an accident.

To control bleeding in the mouth

1. Remove broken teeth, dentures, and any dirt or other foreign matter in the mouth.
Sit the person up leaning slightly forward so that blood and saliva can drain from his mouth. This keeps the breathing passages clear and prevents nausea and vomiting associated with swallowing blood.

2. Control bleeding with direct pressure on the injury, using a sterile or clean cloth pad.

a. **Lip**: Grasp the lip with the cloth pad and press on both sides at the site of the injury.

b. **Tongue**: Grasp the tongue with the cloth pad, pull it gently forward, and press from both sides.

c. **Gums**: Press the cloth pad against the bleeding site with one or more fingertips.

d. **Roof of the mouth**: Have the injured person press the cloth pad against the roof of his mouth with his thumb.

e. **Tooth socket**: If a tooth has been knocked out, wrap it in wet sterile (or clean) gauze or cloth and save it. Place a cloth pad on the tooth socket and have the injured person apply pressure by biting down firmly.

   Obtain immediate dental care (via an emergency room, if necessary). Take the wrapped tooth with you for possible reimplantation.

3. Seek medical attention if you cannot control bleeding within fifteen minutes, if the injury is large or gaping and may require stitches, or if the injury was caused by a dirty object or if the person has not had a tetanus shot within 10 years.

Muscle Cramps
& Strains

overview:

Relieve a cramp by stretching and massaging the muscle and by applying heat.

Rest a strained muscle. Apply ice early, heat later on.

Turn immediately to p. 132.

Muscle Cramps

Important—read first:

If muscle cramps occur during exercise on a hot day, treat also for heat exhaustion (see **Exposure to Heat & Cold**, page 110). If muscle cramps occur repeatedly, consult your doctor.

A cramp is a sudden, painful knotting of a muscle. It may occur during exertion, while shifting position in bed, or even at rest.

1. Immediately place the cramped muscle in a stretched position. For a cramp in the calf or the sole of the foot, lean forward, with the foot flat on the floor; this can often catch an early cramp and prevent knotting.

2. With the muscle still stretched, firmly massage out the knot with the heel of your hand.

3. Use a heating pad, a warm bath, a hot-water bottle wrapped in a towel, or warm, wet compresses to provide local heat.

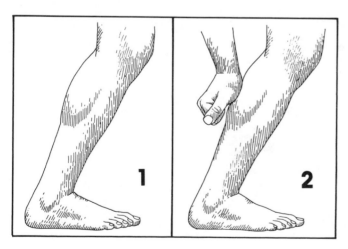

Muscle Strains

Important—read first:

If a strain—especially in the back—is severe, consult a doctor.

A strain, or "pulled muscle," is a sudden, painful stretching or tearing of muscle fibers during exertion. To give relief and promote healing, do the following:

1. Rest the muscles involved. Do not try to "work out" a strain—it will only get worse. With a strained arm or leg muscle, elevate the limb to decrease swelling.

2. Apply cold, wet compresses or ice wrapped in cloth as soon as possible. Continue until the pain subsides or for 24 hours at most.

3. After 24 hours have passed, apply warm, wet compresses.

Doctor's comments:
Elevation and cooling decrease swelling and any bleeding inside the strained muscle. After a day has passed, warmth increases circulation, promoting healing.

Nose Injuries
& Foreign Objects in the Nose

overview:

If an injury to the nose may have broken the nasal bones, control bleeding and swelling, and seek medical attention.

Foreign objects in the nose that cannot be gently blown free should be removed by a doctor.

134 Broken nose

134 Foreign objects in the nose

Nose Injuries
Broken nose

Important—read first:

If bleeding from the nose follows a severe blow to the head (possible skull fracture),
turn immediately to **Head Injuries,** page 120.

For the care of spontaneous nosebleeds (without injury), turn to **Bleeding,** page 42.

Seek medical attention after any severe nose injury.

Broken nasal bones usually produce swelling or bending of the nose, but these obvious signs are not always present. If a broken nose is suspected, do the following:

1. Have the person sit leaning slightly forward so that blood does not run down his throat. Give him a clean cloth soaked in cold water and have him press gently to control bleeding. (You can do the pressing, but the injured person himself will be able to avoid pressure where it hurts). Tell him to spit out blood, as swallowed blood may cause gagging or vomiting.

2. Significant nasal injury usually results in swelling or deformity, bleeding or bruising, tenderness, or an open cut. If one or more of these is present, take the person to a doctor or an emergency room. If bleeding continues while en route, keep him leaning forward and pressing with a cold compress. Do not pack the nose if a fracture is possible.

Definitive treatment of a nasal fracture that is not associated with significant bleeding or deformity may be safely deferred for several days to a week. However, a suspected nasal fracture with a large amount of swelling, deformity, or bleeding should be examined at the time of injury.

Foreign objects in the nose

Important—read first:

Foreign objects are often unrecognized upon visual inspection.

Do not allow the person to inhale through the nose.

Do not put any instrument into the nostril.

Children often put small objects such as beads, nuts, or paper balls, in their nostrils, where they become lodged. Occasionally, this will accidentally happen to an adult. In either case, you should do the following:

1. Reassure the person and tell him to breathe through his mouth. It is especially important to calm a panicky child and to keep him from inhaling through his nose.

2. Have the person blow his nose several times.

3. If this does not dislodge the object (or if a small child cannot blow his nose), do not try to pull the object out with tweezers or other instruments. Instead, seek medical assistance.

Doctor's comments:
Bleeding from the nose after a severe blow to the head (not the nose) may be a sign of a skull fracture and should be treated accordingly.
A broken nose may not be obvious, so after any forceful injury, a doctor should examine the nose. Broken nasal bones will always heal quickly, but they may heal out of alignment. Repositioning, if necessary, will prevent both internal distortion, which can interfere with free breathing, and external distortion, which can affect appearance. Realignment of displaced nasal bones is done after swelling resolves (4 to 8 days).

Doctor's comments:
Breathing in through the nose or accidentally pushing the object with an instrument can move it up the nostril and make removal extremely difficult.

Poisoning &
Drug Overdose

overview:

Dilute all swallowed poisons and drugs at once. Then call your local Poison Control Center to find out whether or not to induce vomiting. Seek medical attention immediately while preventing panic and shock, watching for breathing problems, and caring for convulsions if they occur.

A rescue from smoke, gas, or fume hazards must be rapid but cautious. Give artificial respiration if necessary, and if you are trained in CPR. Care for any chemical burns, and watch for signs of shock.

136-137 Swallowed poisons & drugs

138 Inhaled poisons—rescue & treatment

Poisoning & Drug Overdose
Swallowed poisons & drugs

Important—read first:

Know the telephone number of your local poison control center. In case of poisoning, **call your local poison control center first.** You should have this telephone number handy. You can look it up in your local telephone book.

If you don't have the number, dial 911 or Operator. If there is no Poison Control Center in your area, call the nearest hospital emergency room or your doctor. Tell them:

- ☐ The kind of poison swallowed
- ☐ How much was swallowed
- ☐ When it was swallowed
- ☐ The person's age
- ☐ His symptoms, if any
- ☐ Whether or not he has vomited
- ☐ What you have given him to drink
- ☐ How long it will take you to reach an emergency room

The Poison Control Center will tell you whether or not to induce vomiting. They may recommend using activated charcoal, epsom salts, or specific neutralizing products in certain circumstances.

Always follow the instructions given by a Poison Control Center.

Do not induce vomiting if the poison could be a strong acid or alkali (corrosive) or a petroleum-like product—unless you are instructed to do so by a Poison Control Center.

Do not try to neutralize swallowed poison unless instructed to do so by a Poison Control Center.

Do not trust antidote information on product labels.

Do not use mustard or salt to induce vomiting.

If the person is unconscious and having convulsions, do not induce vomiting or give him liquids. Contact medical help immediately.

If convulsions occur, do not put anything in the person's mouth, including your fingers.

After giving first aid, seek medical attention immediately. Take with you to the emergency room the poison container, any leftover medication or drugs, the poisonous plant or spoiled food, and any vomited material.

When poisoning or drug abuse has occurred or is suspected, act quickly—don't wait for symptoms to develop.

If the person is vomiting, unconscious, or having convulsions **OR** if you think he is withdrawing from a drug to which he is addicted, go directly to Step 3.

In all other cases, start with Step 1.

First aid for swallowed poisons

1. Call your local Poison Control Center. If you cannot reach an authoritative source of advice, you must decide on your own whether or not to induce vomiting. If the person is unconscious or losing consciousness, do not induce vomiting. Look at the information on the product label: If a strong acid, alkali, or petroleum-like substance was swallowed, do not induce vomiting. The following lists will help you. **If you are unsure about what the person has swallowed, do not make the person vomit.**

Doctor's comments:
The fastest way to remove swallowed poisons from the body is to induce vomiting, but this is dangerous in two situations: (1) Acids and alkalis burn the mouth and throat when they are swallowed, and they can produce more burning when they are vomited up. (2) Petroleum-like products give off fumes that can cause a severe type of pneumonia and may be inhaled during vomiting. In general, avoid vomiting up these substances—but check with a Poison Control Center. With specific information on the person's age and symptoms, the type of poison and the amount and time taken, poison experts can weigh the exact risks involved. Do whatever they suggest.

A Poison Control Center is the best source of rapid and accurate information. Many hospital emergency rooms and most doctors do not have information that is as complete or as easy to locate.

Emergency and antidote directions on containers of household products and other poisonous materials are often inaccurate or out-of-date and cannot be relied on.

Withdrawal after prolonged use of alcohol and other drugs can produce symptoms that are just as severe as those caused by acute overdoses. In both cases, first aid and immediate medical care are equally important. During drug withdrawal, it is even more essential to provide reassurance and to keep the person calm.

Pesticides are commonly found around the home. They are poisonous not only if swallowed but also if inhaled or absorbed by the skin. Remove persons who have inhaled pesticides to fresh air. If they have had skin contact, remove contaminated clothing (especially leather) and wash the area twice with soap and water.

This list contains common household products which are poisons. They should be stored in a safe place, away from children. If someone swallows any of these, call your poison control center and tell them the ingredients on the product label. If you cannot reach help:

DO induce vomiting if the person has swallowed:

☐ Most medicines
☐ Most drugs
☐ Any plant part (berry, leaf, flower, mushroom)
☐ Any spoiled food
☐ Alcohol
☐ Antifreeze (polyethylene glycol)
☐ Cosmetics
☐ Deodorant
☐ Detergent (except dish-washer granules)
☐ Ink
☐ Matches
☐ Mothballs
☐ Nail polish or remover
☐ Perfume
☐ Peroxide
☐ Rat or mouse poison
☐ Suntan lotion

DO NOT induce vomiting if the person has swallowed:

☐ Any strong **acid** or **alkali.** These often cause burns of the face, mouth, and throat and include:
  • Ammonia
  • Bleach
  • Clinitest tablets (pills diabetics use to test their urine)
  • Corn & wart removers
  • Dishwasher detergent
  • Drain & toilet cleaners
  • Lye
  • Metal cleaner
  • Oven cleaner
  • Quicklime
  • Rust remover

☐ Any **petroleum-like** product. These often give a gasoline-like odor to the breath and include:
  • Floor polish & wax
  • Furniture polish & wax
  • Gasoline
  • Kerosene
  • Lighter fluid
  • Liquid naphtha
  • Paint thinner
  • Turpentine
  • Wood preservative

2. How to induce vomiting

a. If you decide or are instructed to induce vomiting, use Syrup of Ipecac, 2 tablespoons for an adult, 1 tablespoon for a child under twelve, 2 teaspoons for an infant under one. After the Ipecac, give another glass of water. If the Ipecac does not work in 15 minutes, give a second dose. Do not give a third dose.

b. When the person vomits, be sure his head is lower than his chest so that he does not choke. Have an adult or child lie with his head over the edge of a bed; place an infant across your lap. The person should vomit into a large bowl or pot so that the material can be taken to the hospital for analysis.

3. Seek medical attention immediately—provide necessary information

a. Take the poison container, leftover medication or drugs, the spoiled food, or plant with you to the emergency room for examination or testing. If a plant was involved, take enough for identification: an entire mushroom, a twig with leaves, flowers, and berries.

b. Also take any vomited material. It can be tested for poison. If pills were swallowed, the doctor will want to know how many came back up undigested.

4. Prevent panic and shock

a. While waiting for an ambulance or while driving to the nearest emergency room, keep the person calm and do not let him do anything that might hurt him or others.

b. Have the person lie on his side to keep his airway clear if he vomits. Support his head with a pillow or his arm. If he is unconscious, bending the knee of his top leg will keep him from rolling forward.

c. Cover the person with a blanket or jacket to keep him comfortably warm. If he is lying on a cold surface, also place a blanket under him.

d. Loosen clothing around his neck, such as a tight collar or tie.

5. Watch breathing carefully

If you think the person's breathing has stopped and you are trained in CPR, you can use this technique to resuscitate the person.

6. Care for a convulsion

a. Do not restrain a convulsing person or put anything in his mouth, including your fingers.

b. Clear away furniture and all hard or sharp objects that may cause injury. Move the person only if he is near a fireplace, stairway, glass door, or other danger.

c. In the unusual case where breathing does not start again by itself after the convulsion, open the person's mouth, pull his tongue forward, wipe out any vomit, and give artificial respiration if you are trained in CPR.

d. After the seizure stops, return the person to the position shown in Step 4 (lying on his side). Do not let him walk. He will probably want to sleep; let him. Don't be alarmed if there is loud snoring. Check carefully for injuries such as cuts and broken bones, and continue to watch for breathing problems.

Poisoning & Drug Overdose

Inhaled poisons—rescue & treatment

Important—read first:

Do not light a match, turn on a light switch, or produce a flame or spark in any other way in the presence of gas or fumes.

If you think that breathing has stopped and you are trained in CPR, give CPR **after** reaching fresh air.

Seek medical attention immediately.

Rescue from smoke, gas, or chemical fumes

1. If you are alone, first call for help before attempting a rescue. If you should be overcome yourself, you'll be glad someone else is there.

2. Before entering the area, take several deep breaths of fresh air. Then inhale deeply and hold your breath as you go in.

3. If smoke or fumes are visible in the upper part of the room, stay below them. If automobile exhaust or other heavy fumes are visible near the floor, keep your head above them.

4. Remove the person from the area immediately. Do not attempt any other first aid until you are in the fresh air.

First aid for inhaled poisons

1. Check the person's breathing. If it seems to have stopped, and you are trained in CPR, you can try to resuscitate the person.

2. Check the person's eyes and skin for chemical burns. If there are any, flush the eyes or skin thoroughly with water, then see **Eye Injuries,** page 107, or **Chemical Burns,** page 74.

3. Seek medical attention immediately, even if the person appears to have recovered completely.

4. While waiting for an ambulance or while driving to the nearest emergency room, cover the person to keep him comfortably warm. If he is lying on a cold surface, also place a blanket under him. Loosen clothing around his neck such as a tight collar or tie. Position him to prevent shock:

a. If he is having difficulty breathing, have him lie on his back with his head and chest slightly elevated.
   OR

b. If he is unconscious or vomiting, have him lie on his side to keep his airway open. Support his head with a pillow. Bending the knee of his top leg will keep him from rolling forward.
   OR

c. If he is conscious, breathing well and not vomiting, have him lie on his back with his legs elevated 8 to 12 inches.

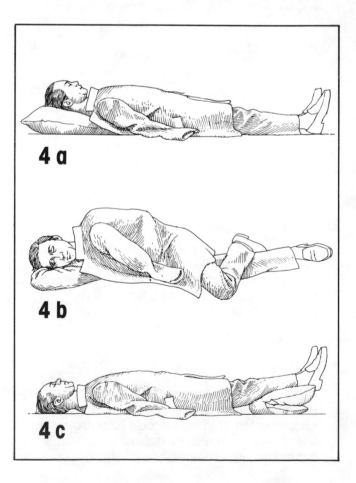

4 a

4 b

4 c

Doctor's comments:

Inhaled poisons include smoke (often from minor stove-top fires), carbon monoxide from an automobile or a malfunctioning home heating system, gases used in stoves and appliances in homes and recreational vehicles, and fumes from paints, solvents, and industrial processes.

The effects of inhaled smoke, gas, and fumes may not be evident immediately. A thorough medical examination is necessary, and a period of observation in a hospital may be called for.

Pregnancy
Complications

140 Signs & treatment

overview:

Several problems that occasionally develop during pregnancy require immediate medical attention. Know their danger signs and the first-aid procedures to follow while awaiting medical assistance.

Pregnancy Complications
Signs & treatment

Important—read first:

Consult a doctor for any injury, serious illness, or unexplained symptom that occurs during pregnancy.

If a pregnant woman partially passes clots or tissue, they should never be pulled from the vagina.

The normal developing fetus is extremely well protected against illness and injury. But, to be on the safe side, a pregnant woman should consult her doctor or midwife whenever any injury or serious illness occurs.

Sometimes, complications occur that are directly connected with the pregnancy. It is important to know the danger signs, which can appear during pregnancy or in any woman of child-bearing age who has missed a menstrual period and may be pregnant. The causes of these complications vary, but first aid takes one of three forms, as described in the chart at right.

Signs of pregnancy problems and how to treat them

If one or more of these signs appear during pregnancy (or possible pregnancy),...	Do the following:
□ Mild vaginal spotting (drops of blood on underclothes) □ Mild abdominal cramps □ Chills and fever □ Sudden weight gain	1. Have the pregnant woman rest in bed, and inform her doctor or midwife.
□ Heavy or continuous bleeding (more than spotting) □ Serious cramps or pain in the lower abdomen, upper abdomen, or shoulder □ Passage of any clots or tissue from the vagina (save the material for examination) □ Fluid leaking from the vagina □ Tender, bloated abdomen □ Sudden weakness □ Signs of shock (weak, rapid pulse; pale or blue skin; perspiration; dull, vacant eyes; enlarged pupils; shallow or irregular breathing)	1. Seek medical attention immediately.
□ Swelling of the face or fingers □ Persistent vomiting □ Severe or persistent headache □ Blurred or dimmed vision, or "spots before the eyes" □ Decreased urination □ Mental confusion and disorientation	1. Seek medical attention immediately. 2. Have the woman lie quietly on her left side while awaiting the ambulance or while en route to the emergency room. 3. Avoid sudden movement and loud noise (tell the ambulance driver not to use siren or flashing lights). 4. Be prepared for a possible convulsion (for first aid, see **Convulsions,** page 94).

Doctor's comments:

Mild, irregular abdominal cramps late in pregnancy may represent "false labor," which is part of the normal stretching process in preparation for childbirth. They do not become regular, stronger, or closer together as true labor pains do.

Mild cramps earlier in pregnancy, particularly if preceded by spotting, could indicate the start of a miscarriage. The condition may subside with bed rest, or medical treatment may be needed, after which pregnancy often continues normally.

Heavy bleeding and severe pain, especially with the passage of tissue or clots, require emergency care for a probable miscarriage (spontaneous abortion), which can lead to shock. A miscarriage is often the result of a defective fetus.

Serious pain and bleeding in early pregnancy can also result from an ectopic, or "tubal," pregnancy, in which the egg has started to grow in one of the fallopian tubes or on the outside of the uterus. Shock is possible, and surgery may be needed. If the involved tube must be removed, the one that is left can still transport eggs for future pregnancies.

Late in pregnancy, sudden weight gain, swelling of the face or hands, persistent vomiting or headache, blurred vision, decreased urine output, and disorientation may be signs of preeclampsia (toxemia of pregnancy), a condition in which the pregnant woman suddenly retains excess fluids. Quiet, gentle treatment and immediate medical care can prevent the major danger in toxemia: severe convulsions.

Rescue
in Emergencies

overview:

If you must rescue an injured or sick person, choose the best method carefully. Some people can be helped to walk; others must be pulled or carried via techniques that are appropriate for one, two, or more rescuers. Stretchers can be improvised.

142-143 Single rescuer

144-145 Two or more rescuers

Rescue in Emergencies
Single rescuer

Important—read first:

In most cases, special help (Emergency Medical Service, fire department) can rescue the victim. Call them first if circumstances allow.

When considering a rescue, do not endanger yourself.

Move the victim only as far as necessary.

When you must move the victim, take the same precautions as you would for suspected back or neck injury (see **Back and Neck Injuries,** page 18).

Do not allow a person to walk if he is in shock or may have a heart attack, a poisonous bite or sting, a frostbitten or burned foot, or a fracture of the pelvis, hip, leg, knee, or foot.

Rescue means moving a victim from immediate hazard to safety. This generally involves special equipment and training. In most cases emergency medical technicians or rescue vehicles (usually from the fire department) can rescue the victim.

Special circumstances from which **you** might have to rescue a victim include fire, smoke, water, electrical hazards, poisonous gases (especially sulfides), and exposure.

When you must move a person, think carefully about the available methods and how they will affect his injuries. Get help if at all possible. Be careful and be gentle.

If you find a person who is dead, call the local police department.

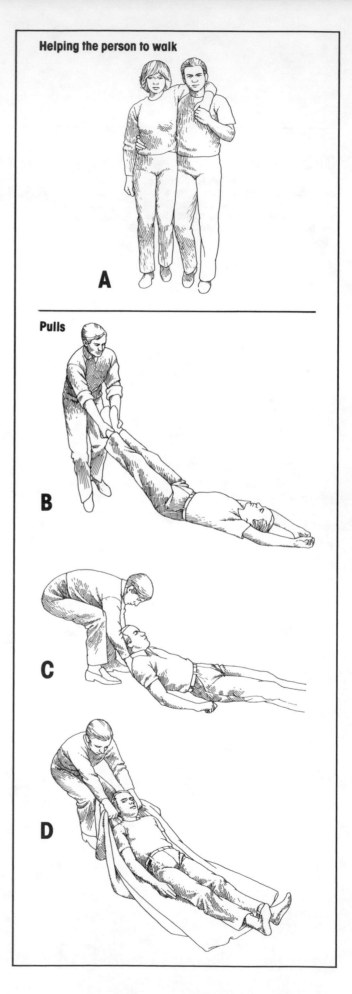

Helping the person to walk

A

Pulls

B

C

D

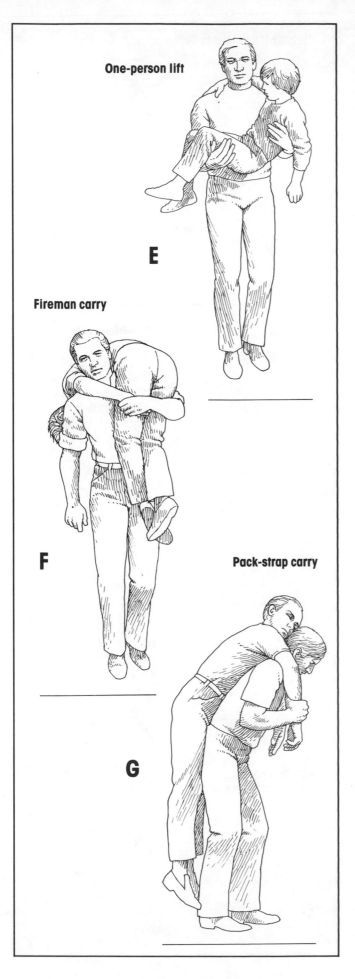

One-person lift

E

Fireman carry

F

Pack-strap carry

G

Helping the person to walk

If a person is conscious and has no signs of shock, heart attack, poisonous bite or sting, frostbitten or burned foot, or a bone or joint injury of the pelvis, hip, leg, knee, or foot, you can safely help him to walk.

A. Put one of the person's arms around your neck. Hold his hand. Place your other arm around his waist.

Pulls and lifts—for short distances:

B. Ankle pull. The fastest method for a short distance on a smooth surface is to pull the person by both ankles.

C. Shoulder pull. For short distances over a rougher surface, pull the person by both shoulders. Stabilize his head with your forearms.

D. Blanket pull. Roll the person onto a blanket, wrap him, and pull from behind his head.

E. One-person lift. A child or light adult can be carried if you place one arm under his knees and one around his upper back.

Carries—for longer distances:

F. Fireman carry. If the person's injuries permit, longer distances can be traveled if you carry the person over your shoulder.

G. Pack-strap carry. When injuries make the fireman carry unsafe, this method is better for longer distances than the one-person lift.

Rescue in Emergencies
Two or more rescuers

Important—read first:

In most cases, special help (Emergency Medical Service, fire department) can rescue the victim. Call them first if circumstances allow.

When considering a rescue, do not endanger yourself.

Move the victim only as far as necessary.

When you must move the victim, take the same precautions as you would for suspected back or neck injury (see **Back and Neck Injuries,** page 18).

Do not allow a person to walk if he is in shock or may have a heart attack, a poisonous bite or sting, a frostbitten or burned foot, or a fracture of the pelvis, hip, leg, knee, or foot.

When you must move a person, think carefully about the available methods and how they will affect his injuries.
Practice on an uninjured person first, if you have time. This is especially helpful if several rescuers need to coordinate their efforts. Be careful and be gentle.

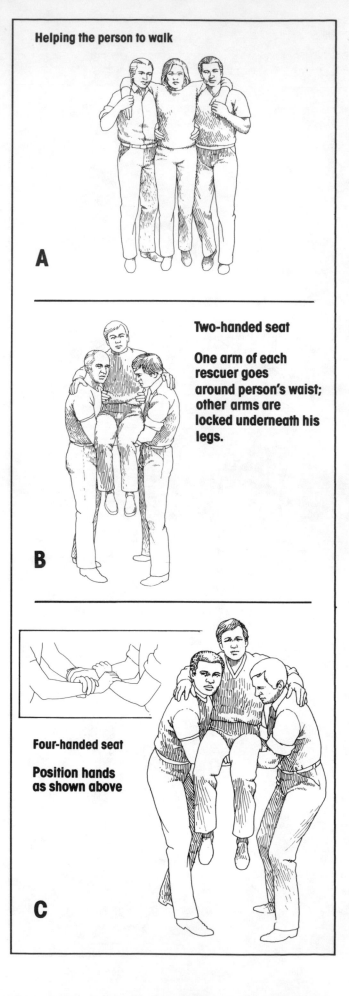

Helping the person to walk

A

Two-handed seat

One arm of each rescuer goes around person's waist; other arms are locked underneath his legs.

B

Four-handed seat

Position hands as shown above

C

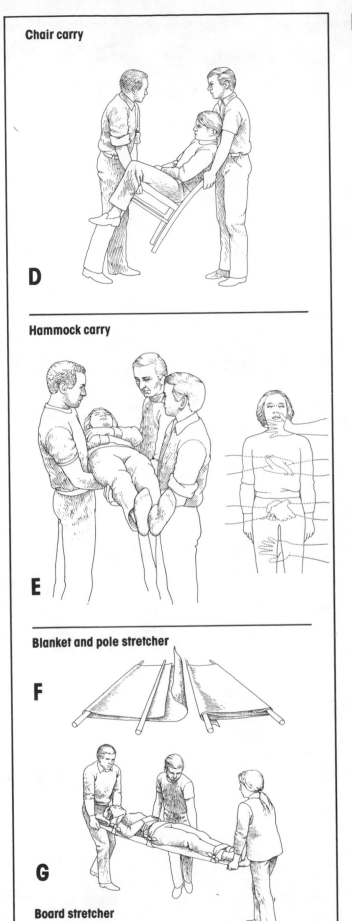

Chair carry

D

Hammock carry

E

Blanket and pole stretcher

F

G

Board stretcher

Helping the person to walk

If a person is conscious and has no signs of shock, heart attack, poisonous bite or sting, frostbitten or burned foot, or bone or joint injury, two rescuers can safely help him to walk.

A. Put one of the person's arms around each rescuer's neck. Hold his hands. The rescuers should place their free arms around his waist.

Carries and seats

Two rescuers can carry a person farther and more comfortably than can one.

B. **Two-handed seat.** This method is safer if the person cannot hold on but is less powerful than the four-handed seat.

C. **Four-handed seat.** When no equipment is available, this is the easiest two-man carry, but it is safe only if the person is conscious and can hold on.

D. **Chair carry.** This is especially useful if the person is most comfortable sitting up. It is also a good method for climbing stairs and negotiating narrow, winding corridors.

Three or more rescuers

The more people you have to share the weight, the farther you can carry a person and the more comfortable he will be.

E. **Hammock carry.** Three to six people stand on alternate sides of the injured person and link hands beneath him.

Improvising stretchers

When two rescuers carry a stretcher, one or two others (if possible) should walk at the sides to share the weight and to keep the person from rolling over.

F. **Blanket and poles.** Oars or other long, fairly straight objects can be used as poles. If the blanket is wrapped as shown, the person's weight will keep it from unwinding.

G. **Board.** A surfboard, door, bench, or ironing board can be used. This is sturdier than a blanket-and-pole stretcher but heavier and less comfortable. It is also easier for the person to roll off it, so tie him on securely.

Skin Problems:
Rashes, blisters & contact poisons

overview:

Try to determine the nature of a rash by examining it and asking about possible causes and related symptoms. Then give the appropriate treatment.

Protect a blister that is not broken, if possible. Drain it only if it is likely to tear. If it is broken, cover it.

Poison ivy, poison oak, and poison sumac rashes should be washed with soap and water, sponged with alcohol and painted with calamine lotion.

148-149   **Rashes (bacterial, fungal, allergies, chemical, heat)**

150   **Blisters**

151   **Skin-contact poisons (poison ivy, poison oak & poison sumac)**

Skin Problems
Rashes (bacterial, fungal, allergies, chemical, heat)

Important—read first:

Seek medical attention immediately if purple or bright red spots appear on the skin. This is not a rash and may indicate a serious disorder.

Seek medical attention immediately for red, swollen patches that enlarge and spread, often with fever and vomiting (possible erysipelas).

Seek medical attention promptly for hives (welts of various sizes and shapes that itch, burn, or sting) and for any rash that occurs while a person is taking medication.

Seek medical attention if any rash becomes infected: The area is tender, throbbing, or swollen, with red streaks leading from it, and pus; often accompanied by swollen glands and/or fever.

The sudden outbreak of a rash can be caused by a number of conditions.

Try to determine the condition in question from the appearance of the rash and by asking about possible causes (medications, contact with irritating substances, allergies, etc.) and other symptoms, such as fever.

Then give the appropriate first aid.

Most rasnes are not medical emergencies. However, any rash associated with high fever, swollen or painful joints, or respiratory difficulty may indicate a serious illness. Seek medical attention immediately in such cases.

Bacterial infections

Erysipelas

Appearance: tender, red, swollen patches that enlarge and spread; often accompanied by fever and vomiting

Cause: streptococcal infection under the skin

First aid: Seek medical attention immediately. Erysipelas can be life-threatening.

Impetigo

Appearance: pus-filled blisters that break and form crusts

Cause: streptococcal infection of the skin surface

First aid: Seek medical attention. Avoid the spread of pus to other parts of the body and to other people. Wash all contaminated clothes, towels, and bedding thoroughly in hot water with bleach.

Fungal infections (ringworm)

Appearance: itchy, scaly, reddish areas that enlarge and may form red rings with pale centers; found most often on the scalp, in the groin, and between the toes

Cause: fungus infecting the skin surface

First aid: Apply nonprescription liquid or ointment preparations for fungus. If they do not work, seek medical attention.

Allergies

Hives

Appearance: welts (bumps) of various sizes and shapes that itch, burn, or sting

Cause: allergy to plants, animals, foods (especially seafood, chocolate, nuts, berries), and other substances

First aid: Seek medical attention promptly.

Drug rash

Appearance: varies

Cause: allergy to internal or external (skin) medications

First aid: Seek medical attention promptly for any rash that occurs while a person is taking a medication, even if he has never been allergic to it before.

Chemical irritation

Appearance: redness and itching, sometimes with blisters or crusts

Cause: irritation caused by a chemical, household product, clothes washed in a new detergent, cosmetics, etc.

First aid: Avoid the suspected substances. Apply cold, wet compresses. If the rash persists and the cause is unknown, see a dermatologist, who can test for the offending substance.

Heat rash (prickly heat)

Appearance: patches of tiny red pinpoints

Cause: blocked sweat glands due to hot, humid weather or fever

First aid: Uncover the area or wear light, loose clothing. Use powder or skin lotion.

Skin Problems
Blisters

Important—read first:

Do not open a blister caused by a burn or by frostbite, or a blister that is part of a rash. For first aid in these cases, see **Burns**, page 69; **Exposure to Heat & Cold**, page 110; **Skin Problems: Rashes**, page 148.

Seek medical attention if a blister is large (more than 1 inch across) or becomes infected.

If a blister is not broken and not in an area where pressure or rubbing is likely to break it, protect it.

If a blister is not broken but is likely to break (as on a hiker's heel or a worker's hand), drain it.

If a blister is broken, cover it.

Protect an unbroken blister

1. Cut holes in several gauze pads by folding each in half and cutting out a semi-circle.

2. Stack the pads on the skin with the holes over the blister.

3. Tape an uncut pad loosely over the top.

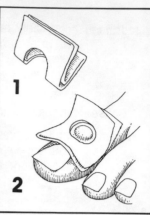

Drain a blister that is likely to break

1. Gently clean the area with soap and water.

2. Sterilize a needle in a flame and let it cool.

3. Puncture the edge of the blister.

4. Using sterile or clean cloth or gauze, gently press all the fluid out of the blister.

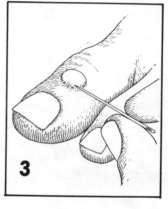

5. Cover the flattened blister with thick sterile or clean cloth or gauze taped in place.

Cover a broken blister

1. Gently clean the area with soap and water.

2. Cover the blister.

a. If it has leaked but no raw skin is exposed, cover the blister with thick sterile or clean cloth or gauze taped in place.
OR

b. If it is torn and raw skin is exposed, protect the blister with a gauze "doughnut" as for an unbroken blister (see above).

Watch for signs of infection

These include tenderness, throbbing, swelling, pus, redness, red streaks leading from the blister, swollen glands, fever. If one or more of these signs develop, seek medical attention.

Doctor's comments:
Blisters are usually caused by repeated friction: a loose shoe rubbing against the heel, a shovel handle or tennis racket rubbing against the palm.
If the blister can be protected and left unbroken, there will be little pain, the fluid in the blister will be absorbed, and healing will be rapid. Torn blisters are more painful and likely to become infected. Draining a blister may increase discomfort, but it lessens the chance that the blister will tear when continued friction is unavoidable.

Skin Problems
Skin-contact poisons (poison ivy, poison oak & poison sumac)

Important—read first:

Do not let the person scratch the rash or touch his eyes or mouth before washing his hands.

If the rash is severe or is on the face or genitals, or if plant parts were chewed or swallowed, seek medical attention immediately.

How to recognize poison ivy, poison oak, and poison sumac

If you think that a plant may be poison ivy, poison oak, or poison sumac, check the descriptions and pictures below.

If you suspect that a rash may be due to one of these plants, check the list of signs below, and treat the rash quickly to stop its spread.

Poison ivy
a small plant, bush, or vine with reddish-green stems and clusters of three shiny, teardrop-shaped leaflets

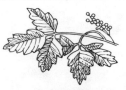

Poison oak
a bush or vine with clusters of three wavy-edged leaflets

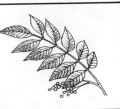

Poison sumac
a bush or tree; leaflets are pointed at both ends and grow opposite each other, with one leaflet at the tip

Signs of poison ivy, poison oak and poison sumac contact

- ☐ Red skin, often with blisters
- ☐ Itching or burning
- ☐ Headache
- ☐ Fever

First aid:

1. Remove all contaminated clothing and set it aside to be thoroughly washed.

2. Thoroughly wash with soap and water the rash and all skin that may have touched the plant.

3. Wipe the skin with cotton balls, a cloth, or a tissue soaked in rubbing alcohol.

4. Paint the rash with calamine lotion to relieve itching and burning.

5. If the rash is severe or is on the face or genitals, or if plant parts were chewed or swallowed, seek medical assistance and be alert for signs of shock or breathing difficulty.

Doctor's comments:
Each of these plants produces an oily substance that irritates the skin of most —but not all—people. Once this oil is on the skin or clothing, it can be spread to other parts of the body. Soap and water remove most of the oil, and alcohol can neutralize the remainder.

Immediate medical care is needed for rashes of the face and mouth, which may cause swelling and interfere with breathing, and for rashes of the genitals, which may cause urinary blockage.

People may gain or lose sensitivity to these plants, so past immunity is not a guarantee of future safety.

Stomach &
Intestinal Problems

overview:

Stomach and intestinal problems are common, but the vast majority are minor. The usual symptoms—pain in the abdomen, vomiting, and diarrhea—can occur separately or in combination.

The first step is to discontinue solid food and give an appropriate nonprescription medication for acid indigestion, nausea, diarrhea, or menstrual cramps. If the condition is mild, this may be all that is necessary.

If the situation seems more severe or does not respond promptly, check for signs of dangerous abdominal conditions, stop all fluids and medications, and seek medical attention.

If an injury to the abdomen has occurred or is suspected, turn to
Bleeding: Internal Bleeding, page 43

154-155 Abdominal pain

156-17 Vomiting

158 Diarrhea

Stomach & Intestinal Problems
Abdominal pain

Important—read first:

Do not give the person solid food, laxatives, or an enema.

If a severe abdominal condition leads to shock (weak, rapid pulse; pale or blue skin; a vacant expression; enlarged pupils; shallow or irregular breathing), seek medical attention immediately.

For injuries to the abdomen, see **Bleeding: Internal Bleeding,** page 43.

Abdominal pain is commonly due to indigestion, intolerance of milk or other foods, swallowed air trapped in the stomach, or menstrual cramps. The person should:

1. Stop eating solid foods.

2. Take an appropriate nonprescription medication for acid indigestion or menstrual cramps.

If there is no relief within an hour, if the pain is severe, or if any of the danger signs described at right are present, stop all fluids and medications immediately and seek medical attention. En route to the emergency room, the person will be most comfortable on his back with his knees bent or, if in shock, with his legs raised and knees bent.

upper abdominal pain

lower right abdominal pain

cramping pain

Doctor's comments:
Young children will often express stomach pain by crying loudly and drawing their knees up toward their chests.

In all serious cases of abdominal pain, see a doctor; hospitalization and surgery may be necessary. Since the most important thing is getting medical assistance quickly, do not spend a lot of time seeking proof of a precise diagnosis.

Danger signs
Seek medical attention immediately

Pain in the upper abdomen, with heavy sweating, nausea, weakness, anxiety, paleness, or shortness of breath. Suspect a heart attack. For first aid, see **Heart Attack & Chest Pain,** page 124.

Pain, starting anywhere in the abdomen, that moves to the lower right part, with tenderness of that area, loss of appetite, fever, nausea or constipation. Suspect appendicitis.

Sharp pain that comes and goes (cramps), with nausea, diarrhea or constipation, or an expanded, firm belly. Suspect intestinal obstruction or a strangulated ("trapped") hernia.

pain early in pregnancy

Pain during the first few months of pregnancy or after a missed or late period, with vaginal bleeding or rapid pulse. Suspect a miscarriage or a tubal pregnancy. For first aid, see **Pregnancy Complications,** page 140.

food poisoning?

Pain—especially among several people who ate the same food—with fever, chills, headache, nausea, vomiting, or diarrhea. Suspect food poisoning; save some of the suspected food for testing. For first aid, see **Poisoning & Drug Overdose,** page 136.

pain after an accident or injury

Pain after a known (or possible) accident or injury to the abdomen. Suspect internal bleeding. Seek medical attention immediately. For first aid, see **Bleeding,** page 43.

Stomach & Intestinal Problems

Vomiting

Vomiting, with or without nausea, is common and usually subsides quickly. It is most often due to overeating, viral infections, or overindulgence in alcohol; it can also occur with allergies, emotional upset, motion sickness, or as a side-effect of many medications. In these instances, treat as described on the opposite page ("For mild vomiting").

Most vomiting is caused by viral illnesses or minor upsets related to foods. This is usually self-limiting, lasting 12 to 36 hours and is not accompanied by fever, chills, severe pain, or blood in the vomitus. Treat as described for "mild vomiting."

Danger signs

Occasionally, vomiting may be due to a serious condition. If vomiting is severe or prolonged, or if it is accompanied by any of the danger signs listed here, stop all fluids and medications, and seek medical attention.

- **Blood or dark, coffee-ground material in the vomit.** Suspect internal bleeding. For first aid, see **Bleeding, page 43.**

- **Severe abdominal pain or fever.** Suspect appendicitis, intestinal obstruction, a strangulated ("trapped") hernia, or food poisoning. If food poisoning is possible, see **Poisoning & Drug Overdose, page 136.**

Other danger signs

Question the person or others involved

- **Recent abdominal or head injury.** Suspect internal injuries. For first aid, see **Bleeding,** page 43.

- **Drug use.** Suspect withdrawal symptoms. For first aid, see **Poisoning & Drug Overdose,** page 136.

- **Vomiting, diarrhea, or cramps in others who have eaten the same food.** Suspect food poisoning; save some of the suspected food for testing. For first aid, see **Poisoning & Drug Overdose,** page 136.

- **Overexertion on a hot day.** Suspect heat exhaustion. For first aid, see **Exposure to Heat & Cold,** page 110.

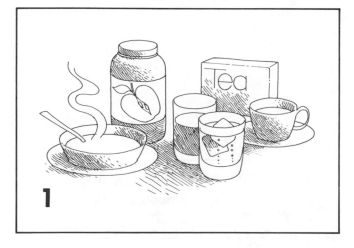

For mild vomiting and no danger signs

1. Replace lost fluids with frequent, small amounts of clear hot or cold liquids, such as carbonated beverages (ginger ale and colas work particularly well), tea, apple juice, or broth. Avoid lukewarm beverages.

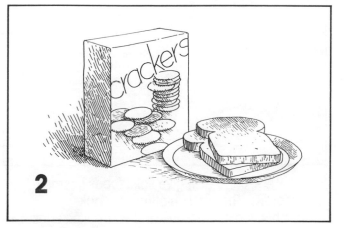

2. When vomiting has stopped, gradually increase the amount of liquid given and slowly add light foods, such as crackers and toast, as tolerated.

Stomach & Intestinal Problems
Diarrhea

Important—read first:

Do not give the person solid foods.

If diarrhea is due to a serious condition and shock occurs (weak, rapid pulse; pale or blue skin; a vacant expression; enlarged pupils; shallow or irregular breathing), seek medical attention immediately.

If diarrhea due to any cause leads to dehydration (dry mouth and skin, failure to urinate, sunken eyes, drowsiness), seek medical attention immediately.

Diarrhea refers to urgent, recurring watery stools.

Diarrhea is common and is usually mild and brief. It can be caused by overeating, spoiled food, allergies, mild viral infections, emotional upset, or alcohol; it is also a frequent side-effect of many medications. In these instances, treat as described at right.

If diarrhea is severe, lasts longer than one day, or is accompanied by any of the danger signs listed here, stop all fluids and medications immediately, and seek medical attention.

Doctor's comments:
During a bout of diarrhea, avoiding solid food allows the intestines to rest, while taking clear fluids replaces water the body has lost. Most attacks of mild diarrhea respond quickly to these steps. Kaopectate is a safe home remedy for diarrhea.

If nausea or vomiting has prevented the person from drinking fluids, dehydration can become a serious complication of diarrhea in both adults and children. With very young children, watch for drowsiness or a weak cry accompanied by dry skin and failure to urinate. Lose no time in seeking medical attention, as dehydration can proceed rapidly, and hospitalization may be necessary to provide intravenous fluids.

Danger signs
Seek medical attention immediately

- **Severe abdominal pain or cramps.** For first aid, see page 154, this chapter.

- **Fever.** For first aid, see **Fever,** page 116.

- **Bloody or dark, tar-like bowel movements.** Suspect internal bleeding. For first aid, see Bleeding, page 43.

For mild diarrhea and no danger signs

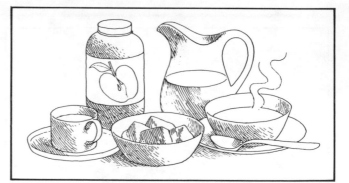

1. Avoid solid foods for a full day and give the person clear liquids, such as tea, water, apple juice, broth, or gelatin desserts.

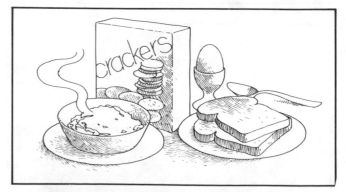

2. On the second day, give solid foods in small amounts. The least irritating are cooked cereals, toast, crackers, and soft-boiled eggs.

Unconsciousness
& Fainting Unrelated to Injury

overview:

Unconsciousness unrelated to injury may be momentary, which is called "fainting," or more prolonged and related to medical problems (e.g. diabetes), drugs, or alcohol abuse.

160 When a person is found unconscious

161 Unrelated to injury

Unconsciousness

When a person is found unconscious

Important—read first:

If you suspect a back or neck injury, do not bend or twist the person's body, neck, or head.

Do not shake or slap the person to wake him.

Do not use stimulants such as smelling salts.

Do not try to give the person anything to drink or throw water on his face.

Seek medical attention immediately. Look for and treat any life-threatening conditions if you are properly trained in CPR.

If you find a person who appears to be unconscious, follow these procedures, in order, without delay.

If you find a person who appears to be unconscious, follow these procedures, in order, without delay.

1. **Confirm unconsciousness**

   Tap firmly on the person's shoulder and shout, "Are you OK?" If there is no response, yell for help—two rescuers are better than one.

2. **Check breathing**

a. Secure the person's airway if you are trained in CPR. Seek medical attention immediately. **Check for injuries.**

b. If unconsciousness is related to injury, see the appropriate sections in this book.

Doctor's comments:
First aid for unconsciousness involves a complex set of competing priorities. Most important must be avoiding hazards to yourself and further damage to the person when there is a spinal injury. Next come the immediate threats of respiratory failure and severe blood loss. Other causes of unconsciousness listed here, while requiring prompt care, are less urgent by comparison.

Fainting
Unrelated to injury

Important—read first:

Do not pour water on the person's face.

Do not use stimulants such as smelling salts.

Do not give the person anything to drink until he has fully recovered.

Seek medical attention if recovery is not complete within 5 minutes.

Fainting may occur suddenly or may be preceded by warning signs, including any or all of the following:

- ☐ Dizziness
- ☐ Nausea
- ☐ Paleness
- ☐ Sweating

When a person appears to be on the verge of fainting

1. Act quickly to prevent a fall.

2. Have him lie on his back and elevate his legs 8–12 inches. (Use this position if the person faints before you can prevent him from doing so.)

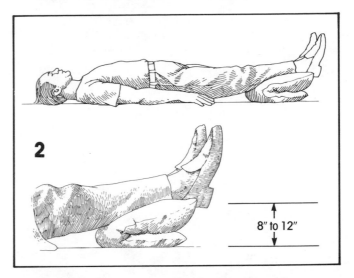

8" to 12"

After positioning a person to prevent fainting OR after fainting has occurred

3. If the person begins to vomit while lying down, turn him onto his side to keep his airway clear. Support his head with a pillow or his arm.

4. **Move hard or sharp objects away to prevent** injury in case fainting represents the beginning of a convulsion. If a convulsion occurs, do not restrain the person or put anything into his mouth, including your fingers. Turn to **Convulsions,** page 94, and follow instructions.

5. Loosen clothing around the person's neck, such as a tight necktie or collar.

6. If cool water is available, wet a cloth and wipe the person's forehead and face.

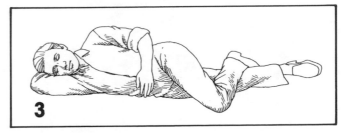

As the person revives

7. Calm him down and reassure him. Don't let him stand until he has fully recovered. Disperse any crowd that could cause him embarrassment.

8. When the person has revived completely, give him something to drink, preferably containing sugar.

Water Accidents:
Water & Ice Rescue

overview:

Water accidents include:

1. diving or falling into shallow water, usually associated with neck injury and requiring special rescue procedures that limit further spinal cord damage;
2. water rescue of a drowning person (non-swimmer) in summer or ice conditions, requiring special training in Red Cross life-saving procedures;
3. near-drowning of a fatigued or stranded swimmer in deep water, or of someone who falls from a boat, which may require training in CPR; and
4. rescue from submersion in cold or icy water, which also could require CPR training.

You may be able to benefit from the information in this chapter if you are trained in CPR and Red Cross lifesaving techniques. Do not attempt water rescue if you cannot swim. Do not attempt CPR unless you have taken a course in cardiopulmonary resuscitation and are properly trained. In cases of rescue after a dive or fall into shallow water assume neck injuries are present and protect the victim from further injuries to his back or neck.

164-165 **Water rescue**
Near-drowning

166-167 **Dives or falls into shallow water**

168-169 **Ice rescue**

170-171 **Resuscitation**

Water Accidents
Water rescue
Near-drowning

Important—read first:

Do not swim to the person and grasp him unless you are trained in lifesaving.

When attempting to rescue a drowning person, always choose the method in which you yourself are safest. Never put yourself in a situation where both of you could drown. Rescuers can drown if they are not properly trained and capable of carrying out the rescue protocol.

Begin first aid for any breathing problem (if you are properly trained in CPR) or possible neck injury while still in the water.

Resuscitation out of the water is carried out in accordance with standard CPR techniques. You should learn CPR by enrolling in classes offered by your local Red Cross.

Water-rescue methods

A. If possible, reach the person from shore with your hand, a pole, a towel, or a rope. Touch him with the object; in his panic, he may not see it.

B. If you can't reach him from the shore, wade closer. Keep a board, cushion, or other floating object between you and the person so that he doesn't grab you.

C. Use a boat if one is available. Have the person hold onto it, if possible, while you row back to shore, or hold onto him while someone else rows. Pull him into the boat only as a last resort.

D. If a light floating object is available, throw it to the person. Do not throw a heavy or hard object, as this could stun him.

E. If you must swim to the person, be sure to take a board or towel for him to hold onto. Don't let him grab you.

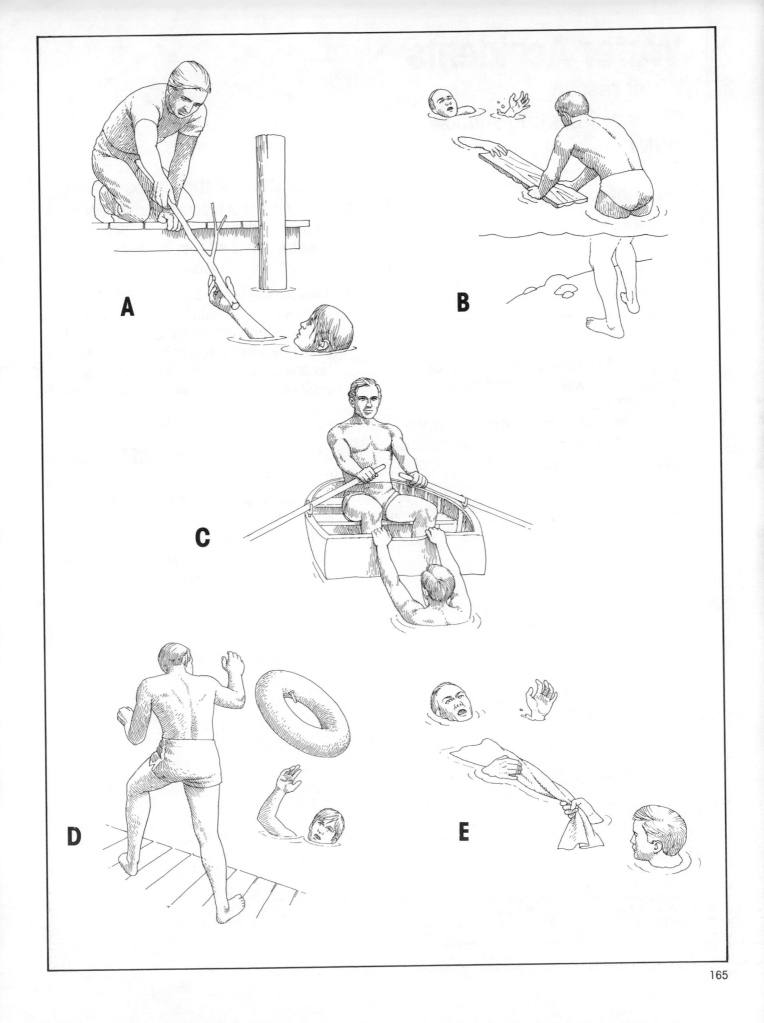

Water Accidents
Water rescue
Dives or falls into shallow water

Important—read first:

Do not bend or turn the person's neck—it could be broken.

Seek medical assistance immediately if the person is unconscious, has difficulty breathing, has neck pain or paralysis, or has been in cold water.

Injury—not drowning—is the foremost consideration when someone dives or falls into shallow water. Assume a neck or back injury in all cases. Do not bend or turn the person's neck. If the person is unconscious, it is probably the result of his injury—not of drowning.

You can use the instructions on the following page if you are trained in CPR techniques.

Immediate first aid in the water

A. If you think that breathing has stopped, begin artificial respiration as soon as possible, while wading or being rowed back to shore. Do not bend the person's neck.

B. If the person is unconscious, paralyzed, or complaining of neck pain, use a long, wide board (surfboard, picnic bench, etc.), if available. Float it under him while he is on his back in the water, and lift him out on it. If you have no board, keep him floating on his back until help arrives.

Continued first aid out of the water

If there is any breathing problem, neck pain, unconsciousness, or paralysis, or if the person was in cold water, have someone call for medical assistance. See **Resuscitation,** page 170, for steps to take once you have the person out of the water.

Doctor's comments:
In water accidents, the first priority is speed in providing support or flotation. Rapid removal from the water should be tempered by two other high priorities: your own safety and the possibility of a neck injury to the victim. Once a person is holding onto a board, a boat, or the side of a pool, there is no need to lift him completely out of the water until you have calmed him and can lift him safely. Pulling him into a boat or lifting him quickly when he is unconscious may make a broken neck worse (neck fractures due to diving accidents are a common cause of drowning).

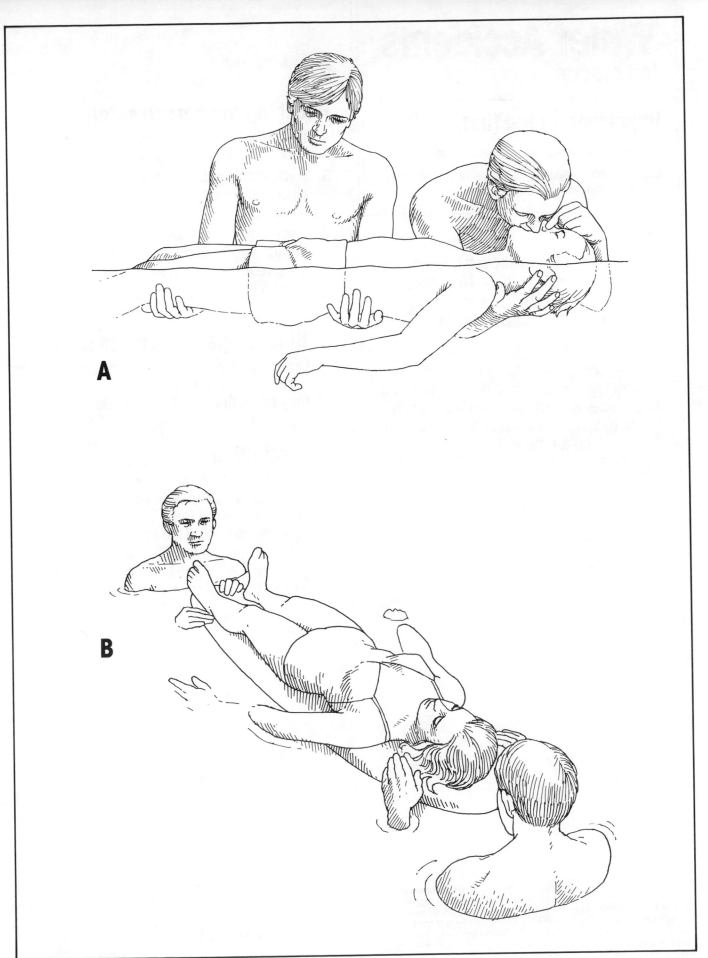

A

B

Water Accidents
Ice rescue

If a person has fallen through thin ice, tell him not to try climbing out. He should support himself with his arms on the ice while you use the safest method to reach him.

Do not give up looking for a person lost in icy water for up to one hour. Immersion in icy water is compatible with complete recovery up to one hour after submersion. Keep looking for the victim while someone else calls for help.

Reaching the person safely

A. If possible, reach the person from shore with your hand, a branch, a scarf, or a rope.

B. If you can't reach him from shore, crawl closer on a ladder or plank held by someone on land.

C. If you have no equipment, form a human chain reaching from the shore. Lie spread-eagled on the ice to distribute your weight.

Getting the person across the ice

Once you have reached the person, slide him to shore on his belly. If he tries to stand, he may break through the ice again.

Resuscitating

Have someone call for medical assistance. See **Resuscitation** on the next page for steps to take, if you are trained in CPR, once you have the person off the ice.

Doctor's comments:
Speed is important when removing a person from frigid water—but so is avoiding panic. If you don't calm the victim, he may break through the ice a second time. If you are too hasty yourself, there could be two people in the water instead of one.

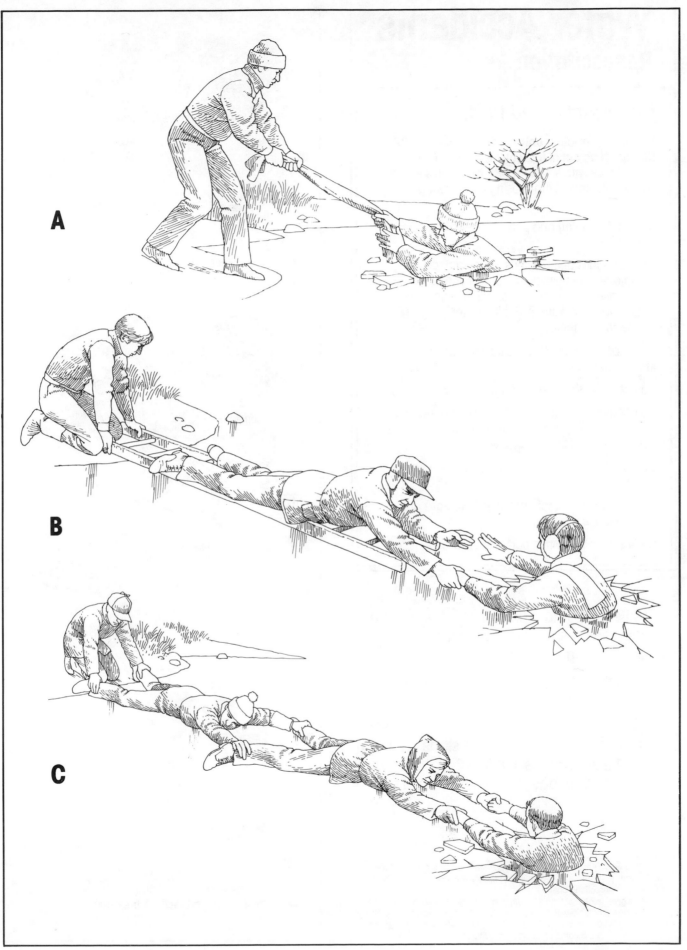

Water Accidents
Resuscitation

Important—read first:

Use this information **only if** you are trained in CPR. Resuscitation out of the water is carried out in accordance with standard CPR techniques which you should know **before** using the following instructions.

Re-start breathing and pulse before doing anything else.

If the person is unconscious, paralyzed, or complaining of neck pain, do not bend or turn his neck while performing resuscitation. If he must be turned over, see **Back & Neck Injuries,** page 18, for the safest method.

Have someone call for medical assistance immediately.

Do not try to empty water from the person's lungs.

Do not give up. Continue CPR until pulse and breathing begin, until exhaustion stops you, or until a professional actually takes your place.

Do not warm the person rapidly with hot water or a heat lamp.

Do not give the person alcoholic beverages or allow him to smoke.

Do not rub a frostbitten part, even with snow.

While removing a person from the water or after getting someone off the ice, do the following:

☐ If you think he is not breathing, re-start breathing with CPR.

OR

☐ If he is breathing, or once he starts breathing, treat for shock, position to promote drainage, and restore body heat.

Doctor's comments:
Do not waste time trying to empty water from a person's lungs: It cannot be done. Instead, perform artificial respiration forcefully enough to blow air through any water in the breathing passages.

Never give up on a person who appears "lifeless" after a cold-water drowning. Low temperatures slow all body processes and sometimes result in prolonged survival. People have revived, without brain damage, after more than 20 minutes under cold water and 3 hours of continuous artificial respiration.

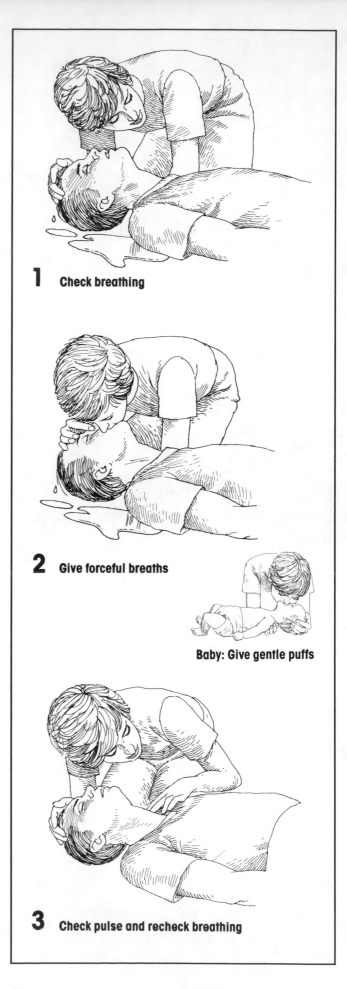

1 Check breathing

2 Give forceful breaths

Baby: Give gentle puffs

3 Check pulse and recheck breathing

Re-start breathing with CPR if you are properly trained

1. Without bending or turning the person's neck, look, listen, and feel for breathing. Place your ear near the person's mouth while you watch his chest.

2. If he is not breathing, pinch his nose closed, cover his open mouth tightly with yours, and give 4 quick, forceful breaths to blow air past any water in his breathing passages and into his lungs. Have someone call for medical assistance, if possible.

   Baby: Cover the baby's mouth and nose with your mouth, and give 4 quick, moderately strong puffs.

Check pulse and recheck breathing

3. Continue with regular CPR. Do not tip the person's head back. When breathing and pulse have been restored, treat for shock and position the person to promote drainage, as described below.

Treat for shock and position for drainage

4. Have the person lie on his side with his head supported on one arm. If he is unconscious, bending his upper leg at the knee will keep him from rolling forward.

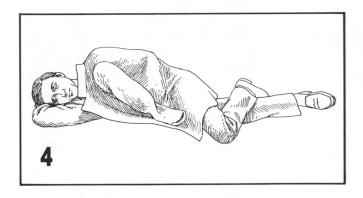

Restore body heat

5. Keep the person warm. If he has been in cold water, treat for possible hypothermia (lowering of body temperature). Take him to a warm room. Remove wet clothing and wrap him in blankets or other heavy insulation. An outer layer of aluminum foil is helpful. If he is conscious, give him any warm, nonalcoholic drink.

6. After the frostbitten part becomes pink and numbness begins to diminish, put sterile or clean gauze or cloth over any blisters (do not break them) and between frostbitten fingers and toes; have the person bend and straighten them repeatedly to aid circulation. Do not let the part refreeze.

Inform the emergency staff

7. When the ambulance arrives or you reach the emergency room, tell the staff whether the person has been in freshwater or saltwater. Treatment differs in each case.

Family emergency chart

Family Member	Allergies	Medical Problems	Medications	Date of Last Tetanus Shot	Phone Number at Work or School

Doctor	For Which Family Member(s)?	Address	Phone Number

Neighbor	Address	Phone Number

Telephone numbers:

Poison Control Center _____

Police _____

Fire Dept _____

Ambulance _____

Closest Drug Store _____

24-hour Drug Store _____

Gas Company _____

Electric Company _____

Dentist _____

24-hour Taxi _____

Other _____

Notes